Table of Contents

June 2017

Preparing to Help

CPR and AED

Assessment

Sudden Injury

Environmental Emergencies

Bites and Stings

Additional Considerations

Additional Information

First Aid Provider

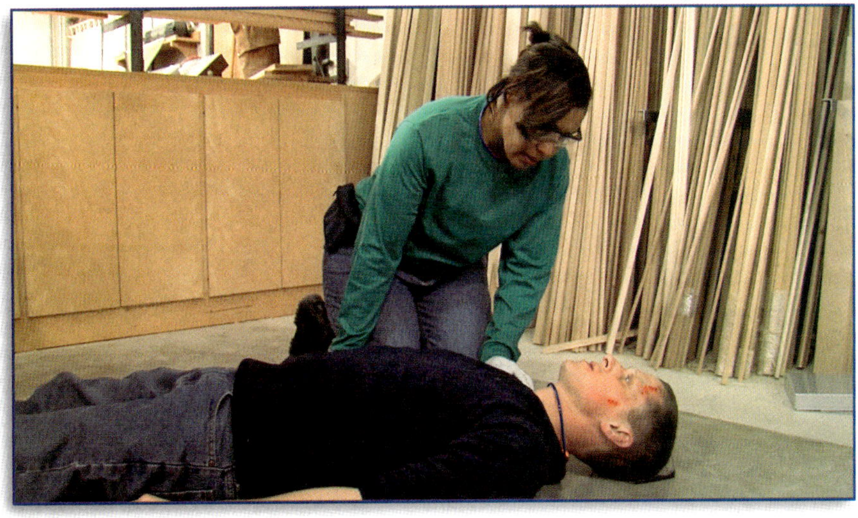

Accidents and emergencies happen anywhere, at any time. According to the Centers for Disease Control and Prevention, there are hundreds of millions of emergency department visits for injuries and illnesses in the United States every year.

Safe practices at work, home, and play can prevent many injuries, illnesses, and deaths. However, once an injury or sudden illness has occurred, effective first aid can often improve recovery and even prevent permanent disability or death.[1]

First Aid

First aid is the initial care provided for an acute illness or injury, when advanced care procedures are not readily available. First aid is intended to preserve life, alleviate suffering, prevent further illness or injury, and promote recovery. First aid can be initiated by anyone in any situation.

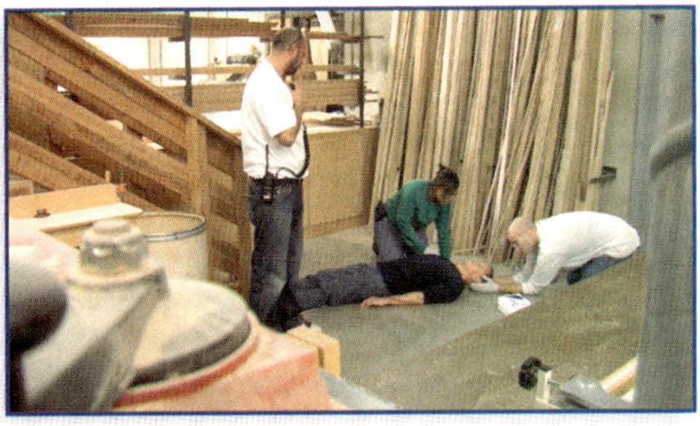

A first aid provider is someone trained to do the following:

- Recognize, assess, and prioritize the need for first aid
- Provide appropriate first aid care
- Recognize limitations
- Seek professional medical assistance when necessary

Recognizing an Emergency

Before helping as a trained first aid provider, you must be able to recognize that a medical emergency exists. Often, emergency situations are unexpected events and can be confusing.

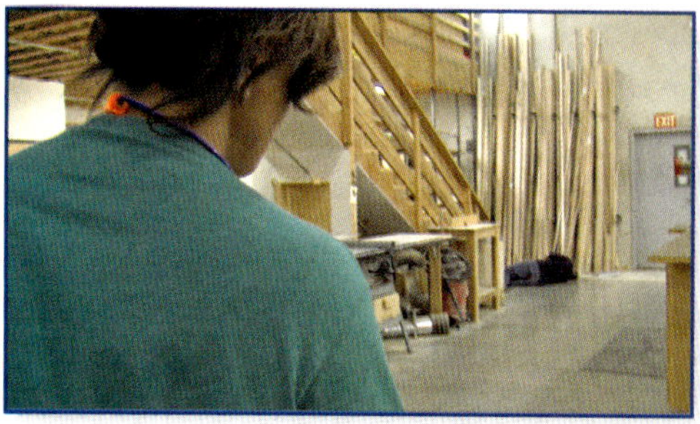

A general impression is a quick sense of what has occurred, or is occurring, when you first observe an emergency scene. This impression can provide important clues to help guide you as you continue:

- Where is the person located?
- How is the person's body positioned?
- Does the person look sick or injured?
- Is it safe for me to be here?

Does the person appear to be unconscious? A person who is not moving and appears to have collapsed could have experienced a sudden cardiac arrest. You could be the person's only chance for survival.

If you suspect an injury, how do you think it happened? Injuries occur due to physical force against the body. The manner in which that force creates an injury is called the mechanism of injury. Mechanisms that transfer significant force are best assumed to result in serious injury until proven otherwise.

Personal Safety

Emergency scenes are often unsafe. Your personal safety is the highest priority, even before the safety of an ill or injured person. Putting yourself in danger to help someone can make the situation worse.

Always pause for a moment before approaching. Look for obvious hazards. Consider the possibility of hidden dangers. If the scene is unsafe, do not approach. If your current location becomes unsafe, get out!

SETUP

SETUP is a mnemonic device that can help you remember the important points of making sure it is safe to provide care:

- Stop — Pause to identify hazards
- Environment — Consider your surroundings
- Traffic — Be careful along roadways
- Unknown Hazards — Consider things that are not apparent
- Personal Safety — Use protective barriers

Deciding to Help

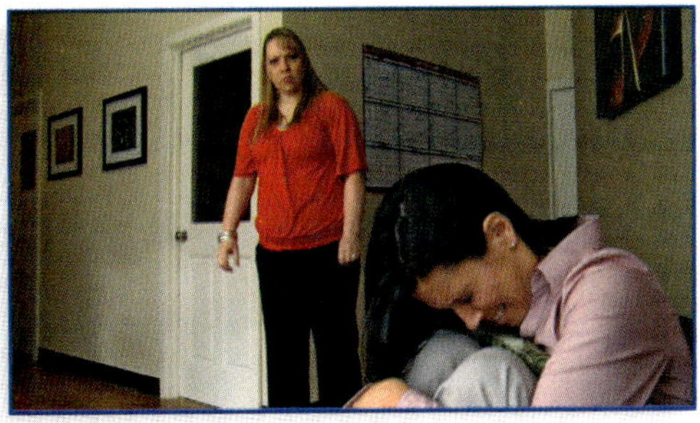

One of the most difficult decisions to make is whether or not to get involved when you think a medical emergency has occurred. It is normal to feel hesitant about your ability to help.

You might hesitate because you feel like the problem is too big for you to handle alone.

- You are only the first link in a progressive chain of emergency care. Your involvement lasts only until relieved by another first aid provider or responding EMS personnel — in most cases, a very short period of time.

You might hesitate for fear of making things worse.

- Your training provides you with sound knowledge and skills designed only to help — and not harm — those in need.

You might hesitate because you think you don't have a lot of medical knowledge.

- Extensive medical knowledge is not necessary. First aid is simple and easy to provide.

Finally, you might hesitate because there are others around who you think might take charge.

- In fact, others may feel the same way, resulting in no one stepping forward to help.

If it is safe to do so, take action. Put what you learn in this program to work. Your actions can help to protect or save a life.

Hybrid and Electric Car Crashes

When involved in a crash, hybrid and electric vehicles have some unique considerations. The biggest concern is accidentally coming into contact with an exposed high voltage wire. These thick wires are colored orange for easy identification. Look for, and stay clear of, these wires. Another concern is the possibility of a vehicle suddenly moving without sound or warning because the electric motor is still engaged. Stay away from the front or back of the vehicle. Place the transmission in park and turn off the vehicle motor as soon as you are able to.

Knowledge Check

You and your coworker are loading boxes into a truck on a busy street when a bicyclist, riding on the sidewalk, suddenly collides into your coworker. The bicyclist rides away, apparently uninjured, but the man who was struck is still holding his abdomen and groaning. You have been trained as a first aid provider and think you can help, but you hesitate because you are unsure about your ability to help. What should you do?

Protecting Yourself

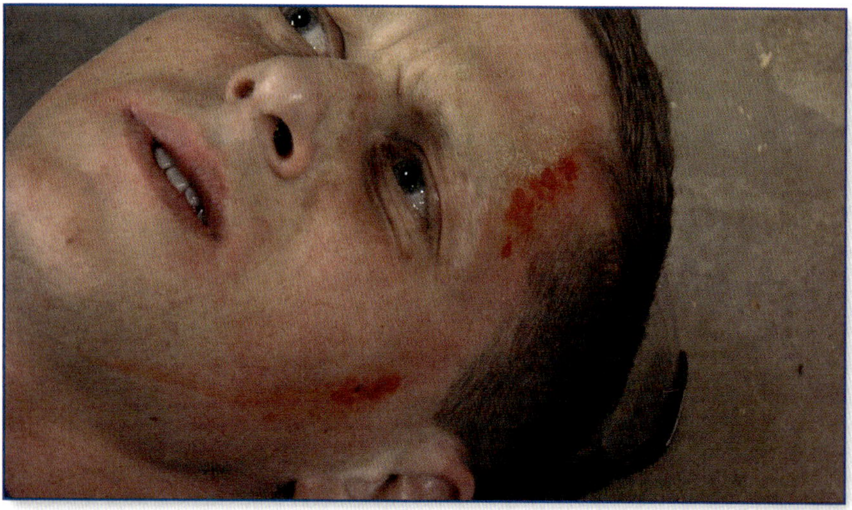

When caring for someone, you can be exposed to blood or other potentially infectious body fluids. While the risk of contracting a disease is very low, it is wise to take simple measures to avoid exposure in the first place.

Infectious Bloodborne Diseases

Infectious bloodborne diseases and pathogens include hepatitis B, hepatitis C, and HIV, the virus that causes AIDS.

Exposure can occur through the direct contact of infectious material with an open wound or sore, or by absorption through the membranes of the mouth, nose, and eyes. Exposure can also occur through a skin puncture with a contaminated, sharp object. Immediately report any exposure to your supervisor. Follow your company's written exposure control plan for additional care and advice.

Standard Precautions

Reducing exposure lowers the chance of infection. Standard precautions is a set of protective practices used whether or not an infection is suspected. To be effective, your approach is the same for everyone, regardless of relationship or age.

OSHA Bloodborne Pathogens Standard

In 1991, the Occupational Safety and Health Administration (OSHA) released the Bloodborne Pathogens Standard to protect workers from the risk of exposure to bloodborne infectious diseases. The standard applies to anyone who has occupational exposure to blood or other potentially infectious materials and provides information on how to reduce the risk of exposure in the workplace.

Employees should review their company's exposure control plan for site-specific information on how to reduce exposure. More information can be found at www.osha.gov and www.cdc.gov.

Personal Protective Equipment

Personal protective equipment (PPE) describes protective barriers worn to prevent exposure to infectious diseases.

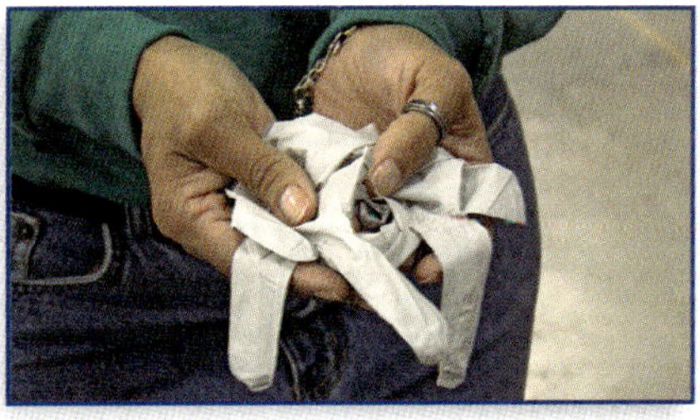

Disposable gloves are the most commonly used protective barrier. Make sure they are readily available, and always use them.

Inspect gloves for damage or tears when you put them on. If damaged, replace them immediately.

After providing care, always remove contaminated gloves carefully.

Even after using gloves, use soap and water to clean your hands and any exposed skin. Use an alcohol-based hand sanitizer if soap and water are not available.

Another commonly used PPE, a face shield, can prevent mouth, nose, and eye exposure when there is a possibility of splashing or spraying.

As an assigned first aid provider, your employer must provide you with PPE at no cost and ensure proper training in its use and care.

Latex Allergy

Natural rubber latex allergy is a serious medical problem. Anyone who uses latex gloves frequently is at risk for developing it. Simple measures such as the use of nonpowdered latex gloves or nonlatex alternatives can stop the development of latex allergy and new cases of sensitization.[2]

Disinfecting Surfaces

Decontaminate all surfaces, equipment, and other contaminated objects as soon as possible. Clean with a detergent and rinse with water. Use a bleach solution of 1/2–3/4 cup household bleach to 1 gallon cool water to disinfect the surface. Spray on the solution and leave it in place for at least 2 minutes before wiping.[3]

Knowledge Check

True or false? You are caring for a coworker who has been injured and is bleeding heavily. Because she is a close friend, it is not important to use personal protective equipment to protect yourself from possible exposure to an infectious disease.

Removing Contaminated Gloves

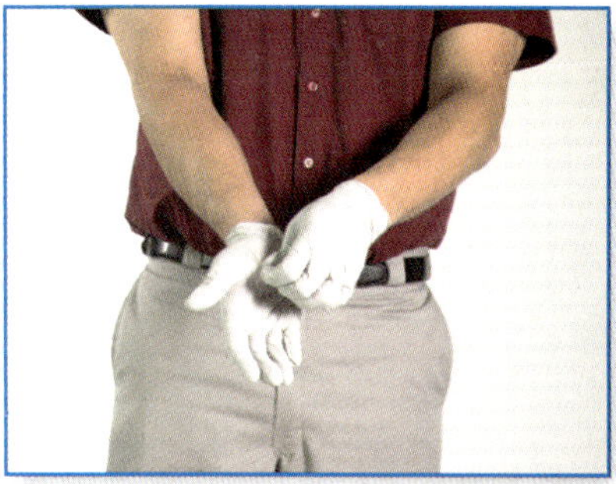

Grasp First Glove

- After providing care, always remove contaminated gloves carefully.
- Avoiding bare skin, pinch the glove at either palm with the gloved fingers of the opposite hand.

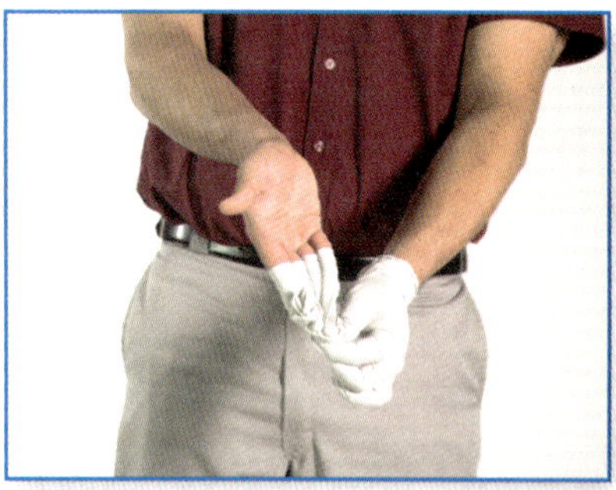

Remove Inside Out

- Gently pull the glove away from the palm and toward the fingers, turning the glove inside out without snapping.
- Gather the glove you just removed with your gloved hand.

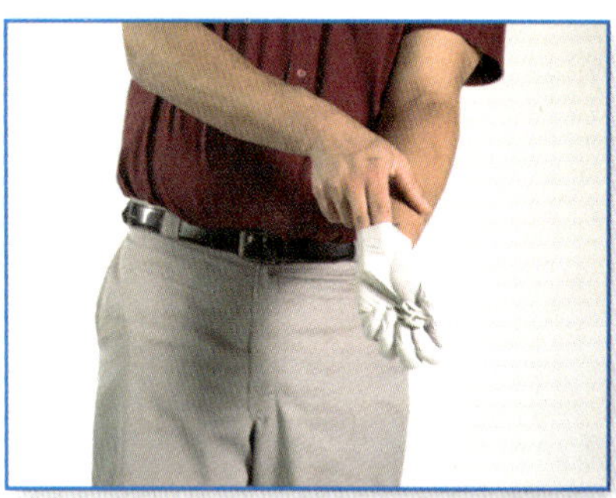

Slide Finger under Second Glove

- Carefully slide your bare index finger inside the wrist band of the gloved hand.

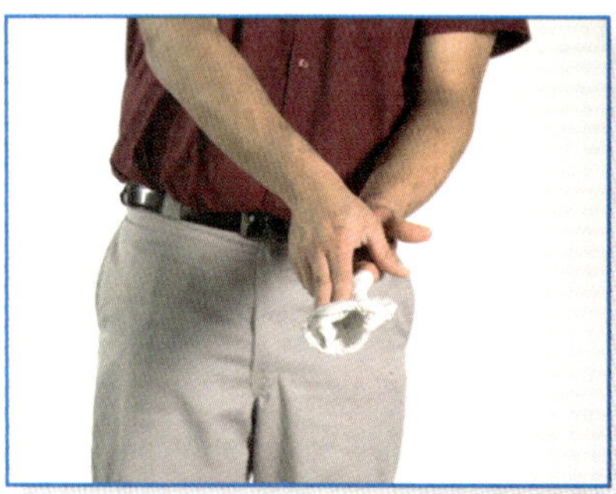

Remove Inside Out

- Gently pull outwards and down, inverting the glove and trapping the first glove inside.
- Throw away gloves in an appropriate container to prevent any further contact.
- Use soap and water to clean your hands and any exposed skin. Use an alcohol-based hand sanitizer if soap and water are not available.

Legal Considerations

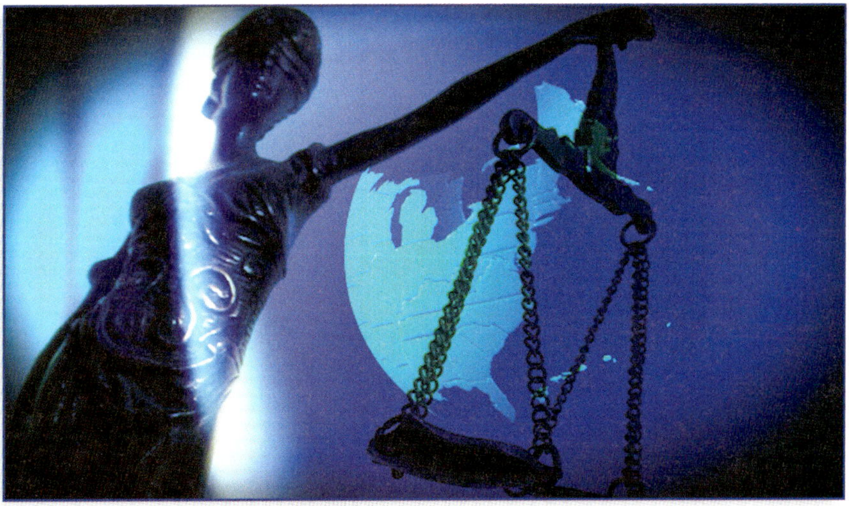

There are some basic legal considerations to be aware of as a first aid provider.

Consent

Everyone has the right to refuse medical treatment. Always ask a responsive person if he or she wants help before providing care.

Implied Consent

When a person is unresponsive, the legal concept of implied consent assumes a person would agree to be helped given the circumstances.

Abandonment

Once first aid care has begun, remain with an ill or injured person until someone with equal or greater emergency medical training takes over. If you are alone, and unable to use a mobile phone, you may need to leave to get help. Return to the person as soon as you can.

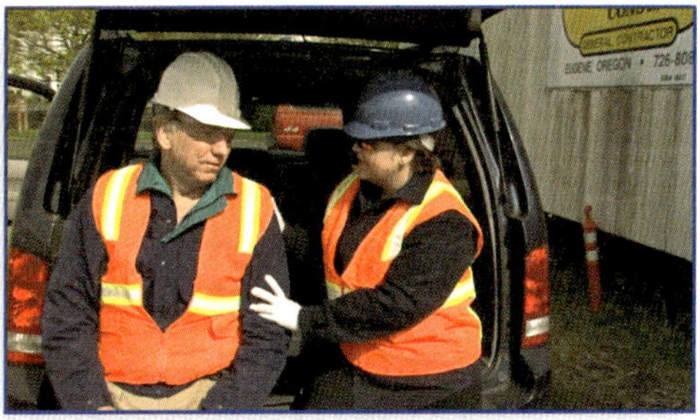

Good Samaritan Laws

Some people fear being sued as a result of incorrectly performing first aid in an emergency. In almost every case, this fear is unwarranted.

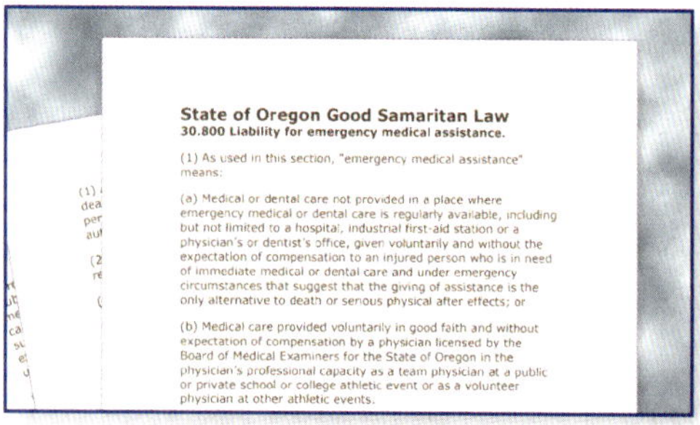

All states have passed what are known as Good Samaritan laws to help encourage bystanders to assist those in need.

These laws help protect anyone who

- voluntarily provides assistance, without expecting or accepting compensation;
- is reasonable and prudent;
- does not provide care beyond the training received; and
- is not grossly negligent, or completely careless, in delivering emergency care.

Good Samaritan laws vary from state to state. Become familiar with the laws in your state and other states where you work or travel.

Regardless of location, it is always appropriate to use common sense.

- Activate EMS or an occupational emergency action plan (EAP) immediately.
- If the scene is unsafe, do not enter!
- Ask a responsive person for permission before giving care.
- Never attempt skills that exceed your training.
- And, once you have started, don't stop until someone with equal or greater training relieves you.

Other Legal Considerations

Duty to Act — A predetermined requirement to provide care, typically by job description (such as firefighter, police officer, or lifeguard) or by relationship (such as parent or guardian). In general, a first aid trained–person is encouraged, but not required by duty, to act.

Negligence — Occurs when someone is caused further harm due to care that did not meet the expected standard of someone with a duty to act.

Assault and Battery — Placing a person in fear of bodily harm. Forcing care on a person against his or her wishes may be considered grounds for this.

Knowledge Check

You return from your lunchbreak to your work area and discover a coworker who appears to have collapsed and does not respond to your voice or touch. You immediately begin to help. What legal concept related to providing first aid care applies in this situation?

Calling For Help

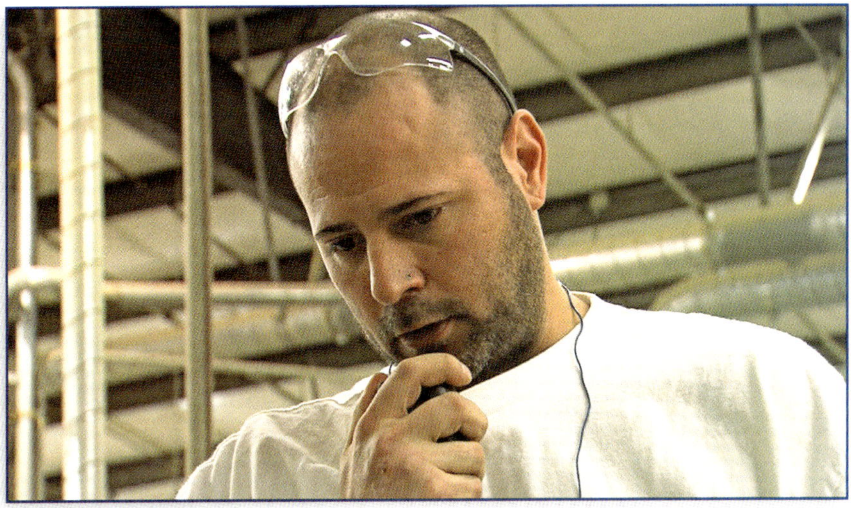

An essential role of the first aid provider is recognizing when additional help is needed and knowing how to get it. This includes learning how and when to activate the EMS system, using the emergency action plan in your workplace, and how to contact your local poison control center.

Emergency Medical Services (EMS)

Emergency medical services (EMS) describes the prehospital emergency medical response system developed within a community. An EMS system uses specialized emergency communication equipment to gather information and dispatch appropriate emergency resources.

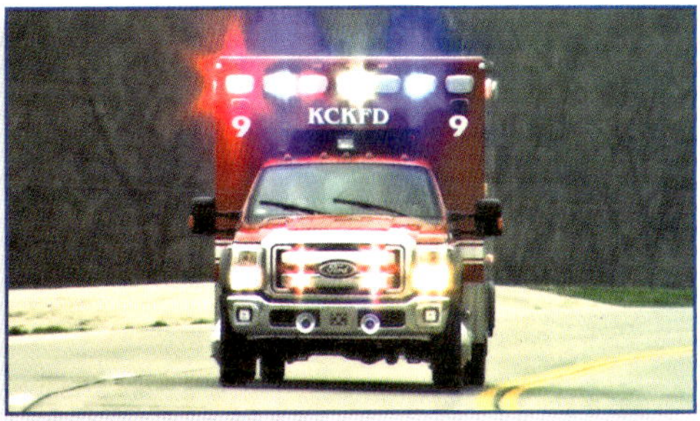

Trained EMS providers within the system respond directly to emergency scenes, provide advanced medical care, and transport ill or injured people to a hospital.

Activating the EMS system usually consists of calling an easy-to-remember emergency number, such as 911. This is appropriate when there are immediate threats to life, a significant mechanism of injury has occurred, warning signs of serious illness exist, or if you are unsure about the severity of a person's condition.

When you make a phone call to activate EMS, a trained dispatcher will guide you through the call. EMS dispatchers may be trained to guide you in the care you provide, especially with CPR.

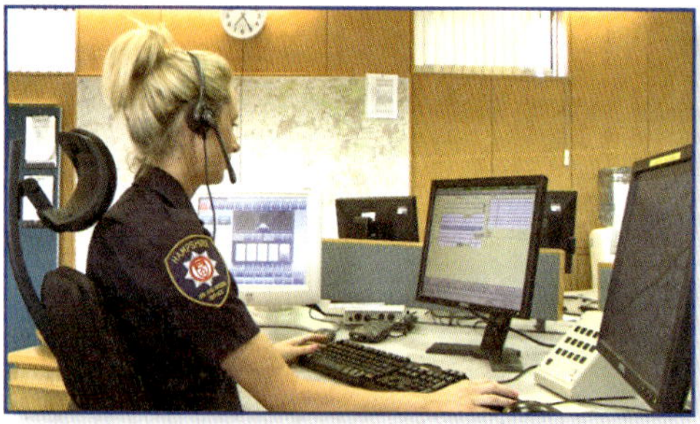

The dispatcher will ask for basic information, such as the type of emergency, location, and what care is being provided. Answer questions as clearly and concisely as you can. Appropriate resources will be notified to respond while you are on the line.

The majority of emergency calls in the United States are now made on mobile phones. With a mobile phone, you can quickly activate EMS while staying in place next to the affected person. The speaker function of a phone allows you to listen to the dispatcher and provide care at the same time.

Emergency Action Plans

An emergency action plan (EAP) is used to help ensure safe and healthy conditions at work. It provides step-by-step procedures on how to report and respond to emergencies.

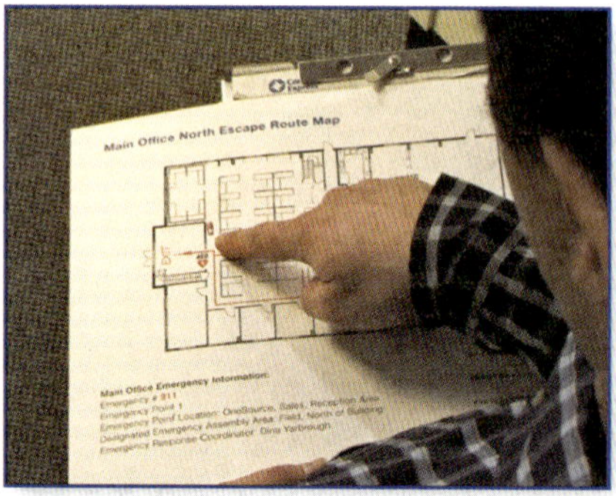

EAPs take into account the specific layout, size, and features of a particular worksite. Almost every business is required to have an EAP.

Emergency Action Plans

In the United States, Occupational Safety and Health Administration (OSHA) regulations require employers to have an emergency action plan (EAP) in writing, kept in the workplace, and available to employees. In a typical workplace, the EAP should contain specific procedures on the following:

- How designated first aid workplace providers are notified to respond
- What is expected of workplace providers when they respond
- How to activate EMS from the worksite
- How to efficiently help EMS get to an ill or injured person

It is important to become familiar with the proper emergency response procedure in your workplace

Activating an EAP may be as simple as dialing 911, or it may be more involved, such as notifying a centralized communications person or activating an in-house emergency team. Make sure you understand your EAP so that you know how to report and respond to emergencies at work.

Medical emergencies also occur at home, so it is smart to develop an EAP for your home and review it frequently with members of your household.

Poison Help Line

Poison control centers offer free, confidential medical advice 24 hours a day, 7 days a week through the national Poison Help line at 1-800-222-1222. This service provides a primary resource for poisoning information and care for suspected poisonings.

Knowledge Check

You enter a warehouse door to get to your work area and discover one of your co-workers alone and looking very ill. After talking to him, you are unsure about what is happening, but you feel it could be serious. Should you activate EMS?

Emergency Moves

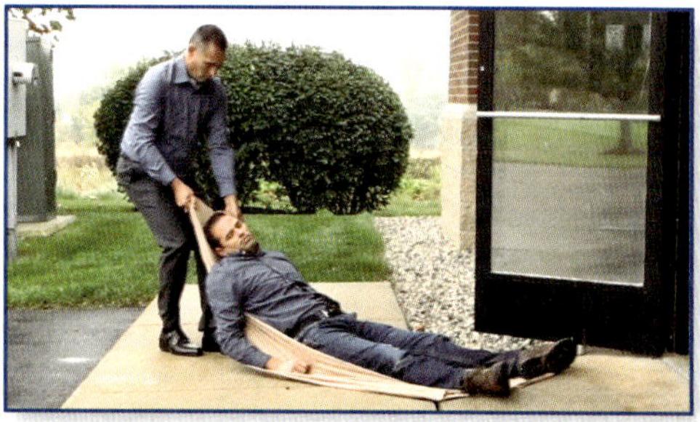

It is best not to move an ill or injured person at all unless he or she is clearly endangered or requires life-supporting care. The greatest concern in moving a seriously injured person is the chance of making existing problems, such as a spinal injury, worse.

If you decide it is necessary to move someone, the most effective move to use is a drag. When using a drag, pull in the direction of the long axis of the body to keep the spine in line. Never pull on a person's head, or pull a person's body sideways.

When moving someone, use your legs, not your back, and keep the person as close to your body as possible. Avoid twisting. Consider the person's weight. Know your physical ability and respect your limitations.

Common drags include the following:

- Extremity drag — grasp and pull on the ankles or forearms
- Clothing drag — pull on a person's shirt in the neck and shoulder area
- Blanket drag — roll the person onto a blanket and drag the blanket

Vehicle fires in traffic crashes are relatively rare. Bystanders have dragged injured people from vehicles in the mistaken belief that the vehicle will catch fire and explode. Moving a person when it is not necessary can make injuries worse. Avoid moving an injured person from a damaged vehicle unless you believe his or her life is clearly in danger.

Knowledge Check

A fire has broken out in the building you are working in, and you are quickly evacuating with other employees. As you exit, you find an employee who has collapsed to the floor and is not moving. Smoke is quickly filling the area you are in. What should you do for the collapsed employee?

Cardiac Arrest

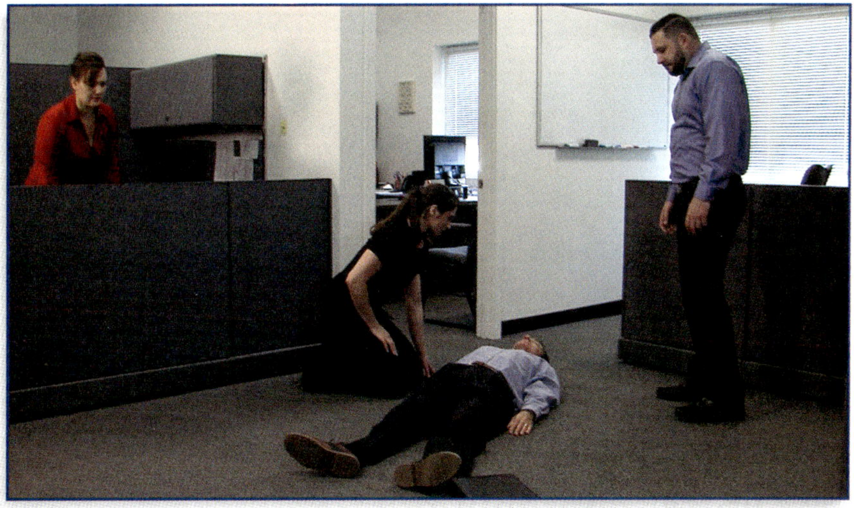

Because the human body cannot store oxygen, it must continually supply tissues and cells with oxygen through the combined actions of the respiratory and circulatory systems.

Oxygen and the Human Body

The respiratory system includes the lungs and the airway, the passage from the mouth and nose to the lungs. Expansion of the chest during breathing causes suction, which pulls outside air containing oxygen through the airway and into the lungs. Relaxation of the chest increases the pressure within and forces used air to be exhaled from the lungs.

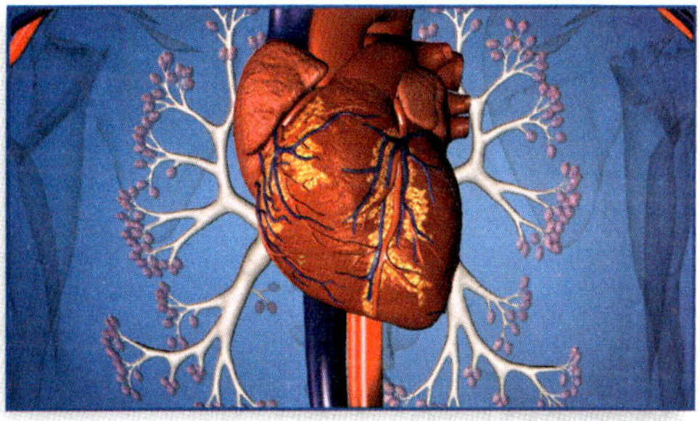

The circulatory system includes the heart and a bodywide network of blood vessels. Electrical impulses stimulate contractions of the heart to create pressure that pushes blood throughout the body. Blood vessels in the lungs absorb oxygen from inhaled air. The oxygen-rich blood goes to the heart, then out to the rest of the body.

Large vessels called arteries carry oxygenated blood away from the heart. Arteries branch down into very small vessels that allow oxygen to be absorbed directly into body cells so it can be used for energy production. Veins return oxygen-poor blood back to the heart and lungs, where the cycle repeats.

The brain is especially sensitive to a lack of oxygen. When oxygen is cut off to the brain, brain cell damage, and death, can occur within a matter of minutes.

Sudden Cardiac Arrest (SCA)

Cardiac arrest is the loss of the heart's ability to pump blood to the body. The most dramatic occurrence, sudden cardiac arrest, can happen with little or no warning. Victims abruptly become unresponsive and collapse. Abnormal gasping can occur. Breathing may stop completely.

The most likely cause of sudden cardiac arrest is an unexpected disruption to the heart's electrical system, in which normally organized electrical pulses within the heart become disorganized and a chaotic quivering condition known as ventricular fibrillation occurs. Blood flow to the body, along with the oxygen it carries, stops. Without blood flow, brain damage occurs rapidly and quickly leads to death.

Cardiopulmonary Resuscitation (CPR)

Cardiopulmonary resuscitation (CPR) is the immediate treatment for a suspected cardiac arrest. CPR allows a bystander to restore limited oxygen to the brain through a combination of chest compressions and rescue breaths. However, CPR alone is not enough.

Early Defibrillation

The most effective way to end fibrillation is defibrillation, using a defibrillator and electrode pads applied to the chest. A controlled electrical shock is sent through the heart to stop ventricular fibrillation, allowing the heart's normal electrical activity to return and restore blood flow.

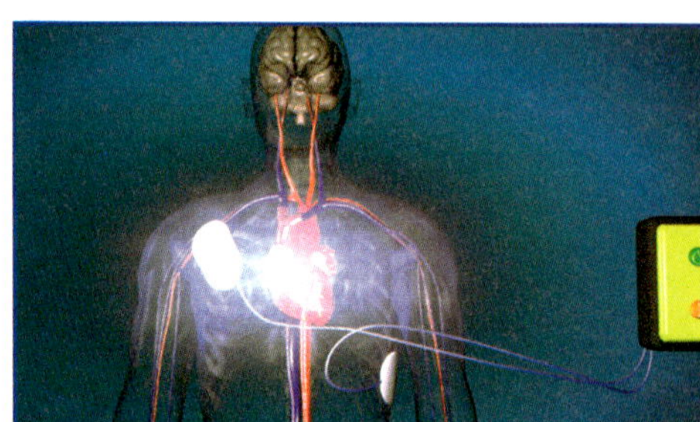

Successful defibrillation is highly dependent on how quickly defibrillation occurs. For each minute in cardiac arrest, the chance of survival goes down by about 10%. After as few as 10 minutes, survival is unlikely.

Simply activating EMS will not help. Even in the best EMS systems, the amount of time it takes from recognition of the arrest to EMS arriving at the side of the injured or ill person is usually longer than 10 minutes.

An automated external defibrillator (AED) is a small, portable, computerized device that is simple for anyone to operate. Bystander use of AEDs has been growing steadily, with common placements of the devices in public locations such as airports and hotels, and workplaces in general.

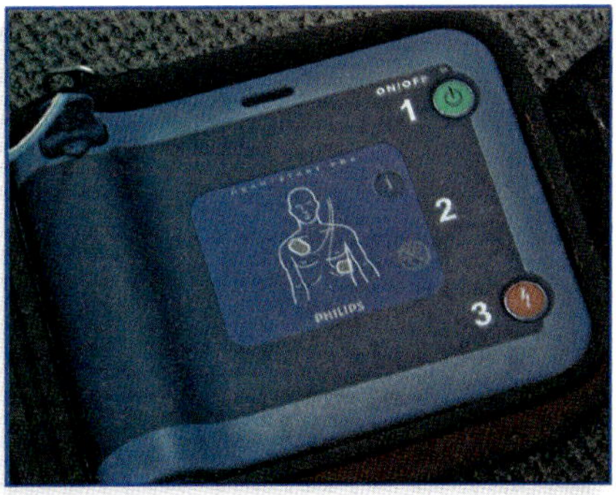

Turning on an AED is as simple as opening a lid or pushing a power button. Once it is on, an AED provides voice instructions to guide you through its attachment and use.

An AED automatically analyzes the heart rhythm, determines if a shock is needed, and charges itself to be ready to defibrillate. An operator simply pushes a button to deliver the shock when prompted by the AED.

Chain of Survival

The chain of survival is often used to describe the best approach for treating sudden cardiac arrest. Each link in the chain is essential for a person to survive. If a single link is weak or missing, the chances for survival are greatly reduced. The greatest chance for survival exists when all the links are strong:

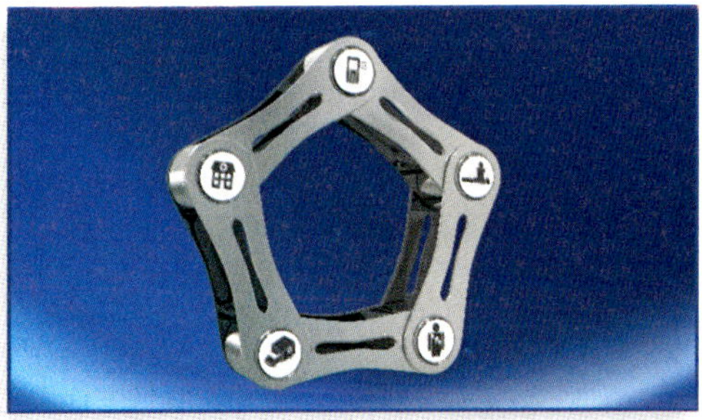

- Early recognition of cardiac arrest and activation of EMS
- Immediate CPR with high-quality chest compressions
- Rapid defibrillation, or electrical shock, to the heart
- Effective basic and advanced EMS care and transport
- Effective post-cardiac arrest care at a hospital

Secondary Cardiac Arrest

Unlike sudden cardiac arrest, in which the heart is the primary problem, cardiac arrest can also be the end result of the loss of an airway or breathing. This is secondary cardiac arrest.

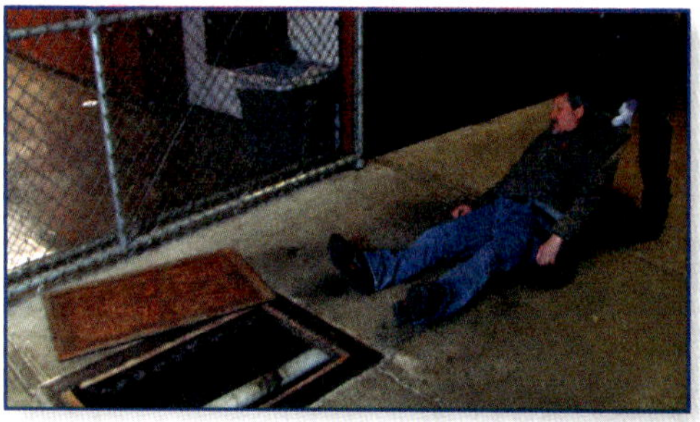

Problems such as hazardous breathing conditions in a confined space, drowning, and drug overdoses can result in secondary cardiac arrest. With no incoming oxygen, the heart progressively becomes weaker until signs of life become difficult or impossible to assess.

If the heart is simply too weak to create obvious signs of life, immediate CPR, with an emphasis on effective rescue breaths, may be the only chance to restore them.

Opioid Overdose

The abuse of opioid drugs to get a euphoric high is a serious and growing health problem. Increasing prescriptions for opioid pain relievers, such as hydrocodone and oxycodone, have made them more commonly available. The use of heroin, a highly addictive opioid, also contributes to the problem.

As a result, the number of overdoses and deaths from prescription opioids and heroin has increased dramatically. Opioids, taken in excess, can depress and stop breathing. Opioid overdose is a clear cause of secondary cardiac arrest.

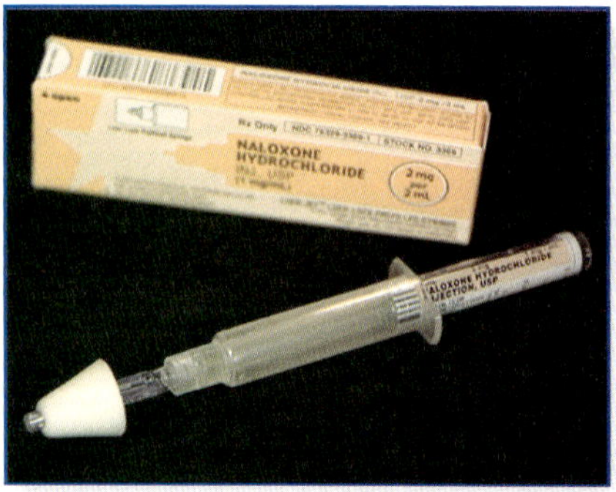

Naloxone, also known as Narcan, is a medication that can temporarily reverse the life-threatening effects of opioids. It is easy to administer, either through an auto-injector device or through an aerosol that is sprayed into the nose. Naloxone is becoming more readily available to lay providers.

It is reasonable to provide education and training on responding to suspected opioid overdoses, including the administration of naloxone, to those most likely to be involved with this type of emergency. Laws regarding first aid administration of naloxone vary by city and state. As with Good Samaritan laws, know the laws in your area.

Knowledge Check

The chain of survival is often used to describe the best approach for treating sudden cardiac arrest. The first three links of the chain are typically the responsibility of a trained first aid provider. Describe those links.

Chest Compressions

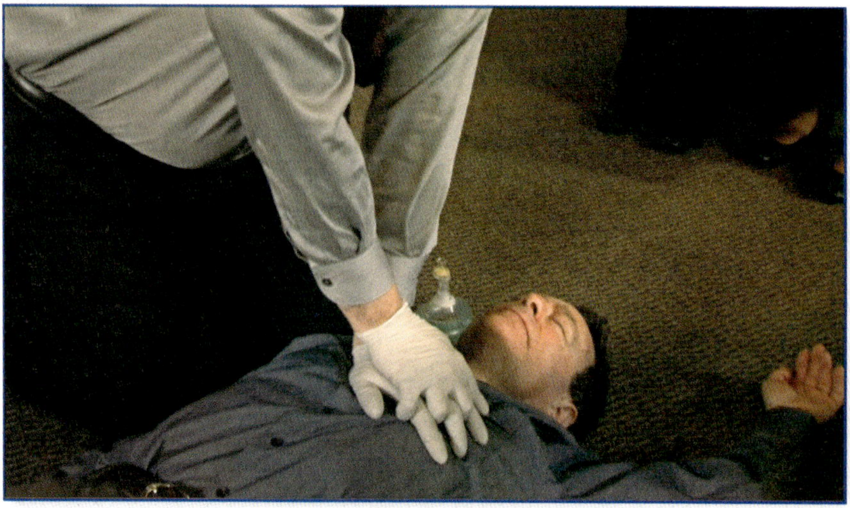

There is a set of basic CPR skills used to provide the most effective approach to cardiac arrest.

External compression of the chest increases pressure inside the chest and directly compresses the heart, forcing blood to move from the chest to the lungs, brain, and the rest of the body.

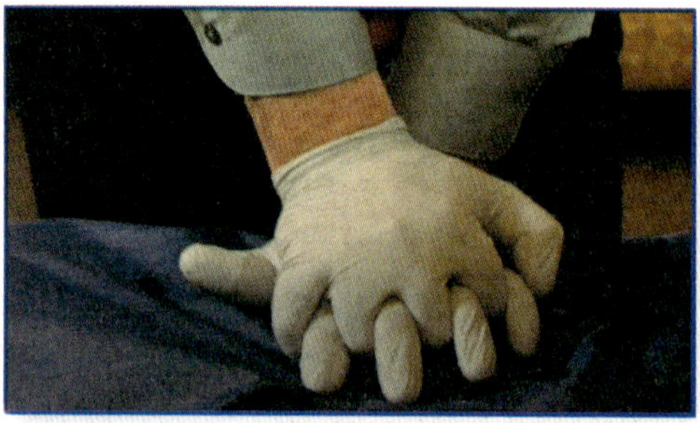

Quality matters. The better you compress, the greater the influence on survival. Focus on high-quality techniques:

- Compress deeply, more than 2 inches. It is likely you will not compress deep enough. While injury could occur from deeper compressions, do not let the fear of this affect compression depth.
- Compress fast, between 100 and 120 times per minute. Do not let a higher compression speed result in shallower compression depth.
- Allow the chest wall to fully recoil, or rebound, between compressions. Avoid leaning on the chest at the top of each compression.

When compressing properly, you may hear and feel changes in the chest wall. This is normal. Forceful external chest compressions may cause chest injury, but are critical if the person is to survive. Reassess your hand positioning and continue compressions.

Knowledge Check

What are the 3 measures of high-quality chest compressions?

Chest Compressions

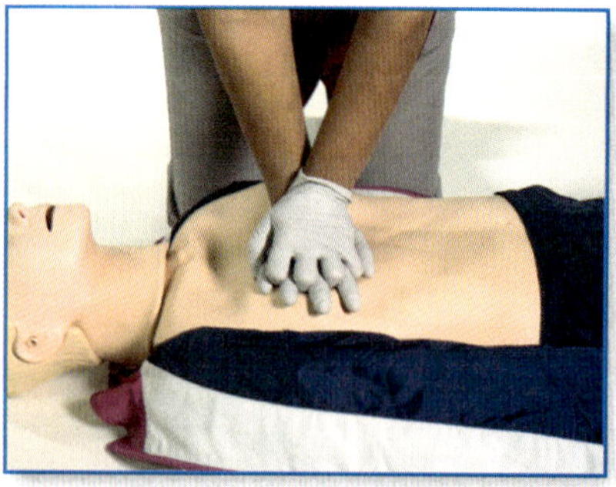

Position Your Hands

- Position person face up on a firm, flat surface. Kneel close to chest.
- Place heel of one hand on center of chest, on lower half of breastbone.
- Place heel of your other hand on top of and parallel to first. You can interlace your fingers to keep them off chest.

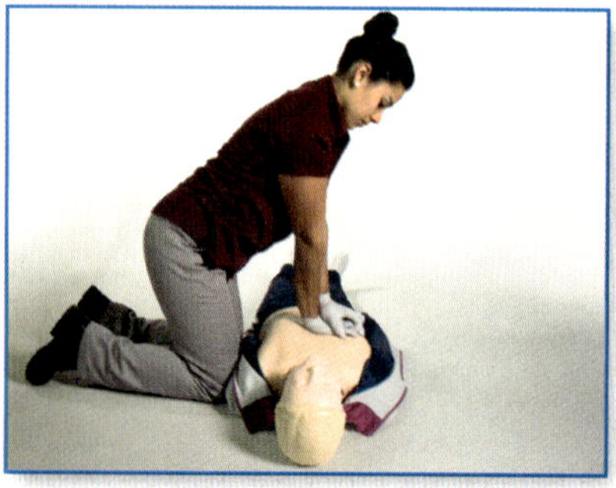

Position Your Body

- Bring your body up and over chest so your shoulders are directly above your hands. Straighten your arms and lock your elbows.

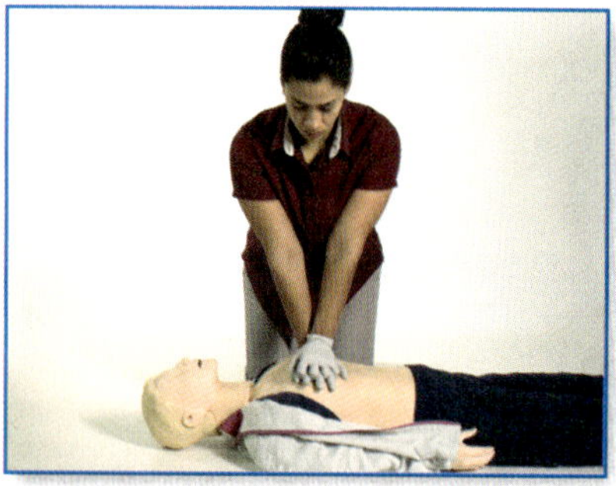

Compress

- Bending at the waist, use upper body weight to push straight down at least 2 inches.
- Lift hands and allow chest to fully return to its normal position. Move immediately into downstroke of next compression.
- Avoid leaning on chest at the top of each compression.
- Continue compressions at a rate of 100–120 times per minute.

Rescue Breaths

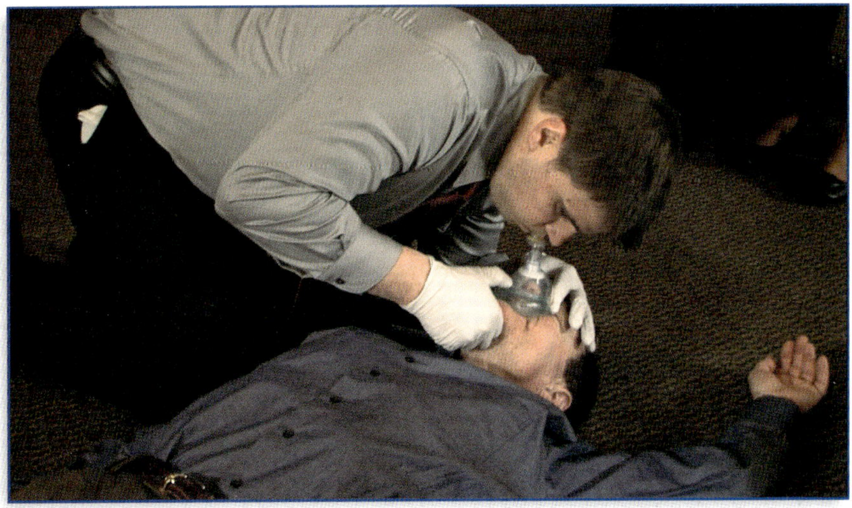

Rescue breaths are artificial breaths given to someone who is not breathing. They are given by blowing air into the mouth to inflate the lungs.

The air you breathe contains about 21% oxygen. Your exhaled air still contains between 16% and 17% oxygen. This exhaled oxygen is enough to support someone's life.

Establishing an Airway

To give rescue breaths, you need to make sure there is an open airway. The airway is the only path for getting air into the lungs.

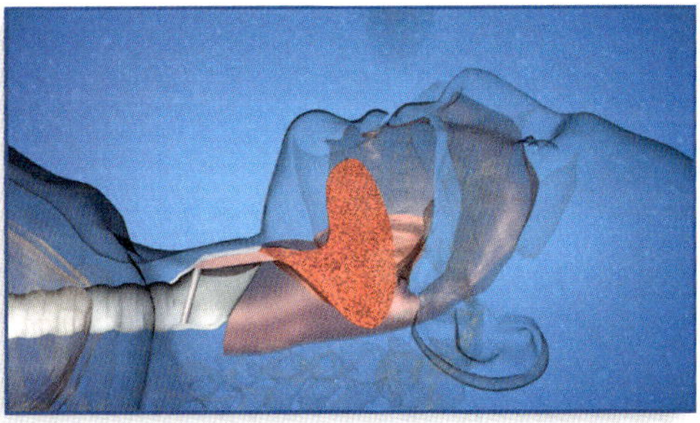

Someone who is unresponsive can lose muscle tone. If flat on his or her back, the base of the tongue can relax and obstruct the airway. This is the most common cause of a blocked airway.

The tongue is attached to the lower jaw. Lifting the jaw forward, while keeping the mouth open, pulls the tongue away from the back of the throat and opens the airway.

You can open a person's airway by using the head tilt-chin lift technique:

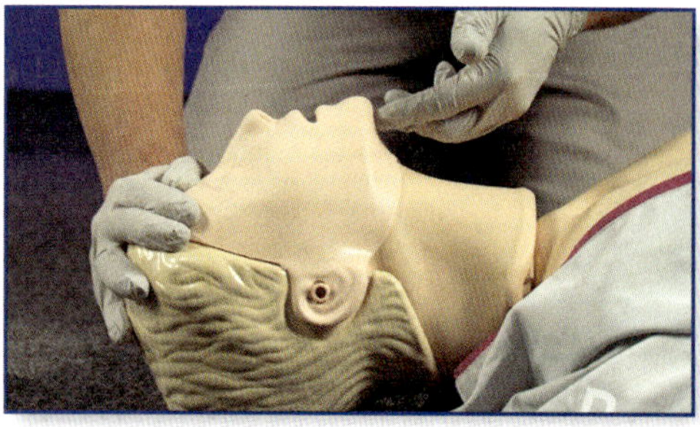

- Place one hand on the forehead.
- Place the fingertips of your other hand under the bony part of the chin.
- Apply firm, backward pressure on the forehead while lifting the chin upward. This will tilt the head back and move the jaw forward.
- Avoid pressing into the soft tissue of the chin with your fingers, as this can also obstruct the airway.
- Leave the mouth slightly open.

When caring for someone who is seriously injured, establishing an open airway is a higher priority than protecting a possible injury to the spine. Without an airway, a person will not survive, regardless of illness or injury.

Using Barrier Devices

As a trained provider, you should use a protective barrier such as a CPR mask or overlay shield when giving rescue breaths, to minimize your exposure to infectious disease.

Delivering Breaths

Each breath should be about 1 second in length and have only enough air to create a visible rise of the chest, but no more. Additional air is unnecessary.

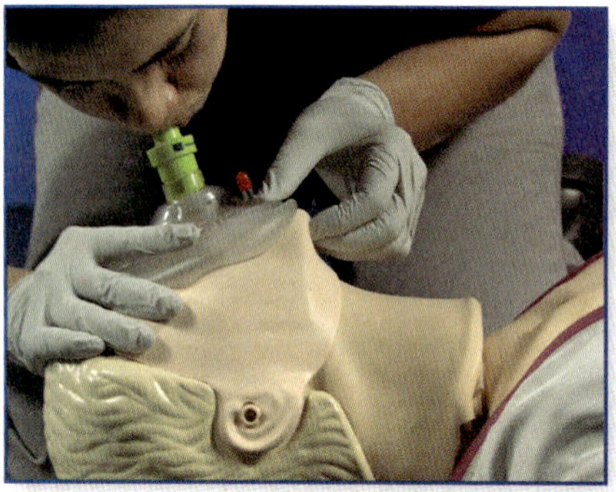

During CPR, 2 rescue breaths are given at a time. Provide these as quickly as you can, in less than 10 seconds.

Remove your mouth and let the person exhale between breaths. Take a regular breath before delivering the 2nd rescue breath.

If you remove your hands from the head, the airway will close again. It is necessary to open the airway each time you give rescue breaths.

If you cannot get the chest to rise with a breath, reposition the head further back by using head tilt-chin lift again, and try another breath.

When giving rescue breaths, avoid blowing too hard or too long. This reduces the quality of your care. Air can be pushed into the stomach, making additional breaths more difficult and increasing the chance of vomiting.

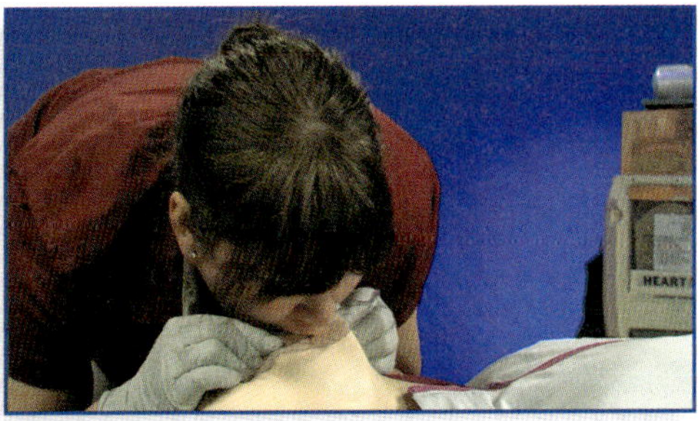

Unprotected Rescue Breaths

A provider may elect not to use barriers, depending on his or her relationship to the person and knowledge of the person's health status. Direct mouth-to-mouth rescue breaths can be performed using the same technique as with an overlay shield.

Mouth-to-nose rescue breaths may be useful if you have difficulty with mouth-to-mouth. Tilt the head back and close the mouth when lifting the chin. Seal your mouth around the nose and blow.

Knowledge Check

What is the recommended length and volume of a rescue breath?

Rescue Breaths — CPR Mask

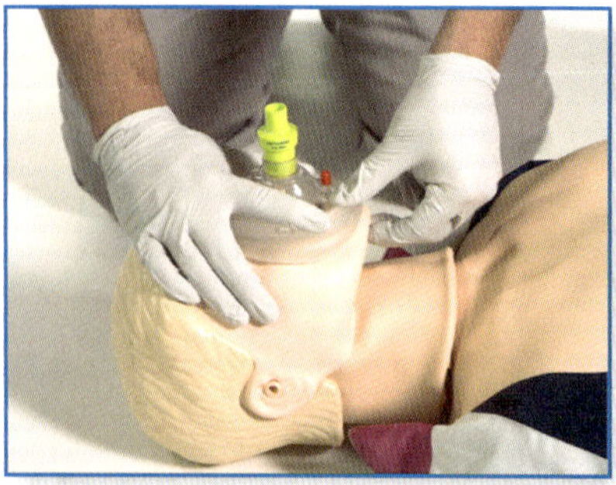

Position Mask

- Inspect mask to make sure one-way valve is in place.
- Place mask flat on person's face with top of mask over bridge of nose.
- Use thumb and forefinger to provide uniform pressure around top of mask.
- Use thumb of your hand lifting chin to control bottom.

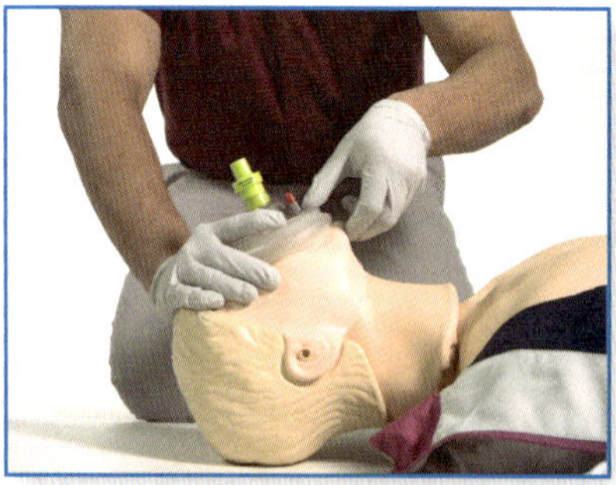

Open Airway

- Hook fingertips of hand controlling bottom of mask under bony ridge of chin.
- Tilt head and lift chin to open airway. Lift face up into mask to create an airtight seal.

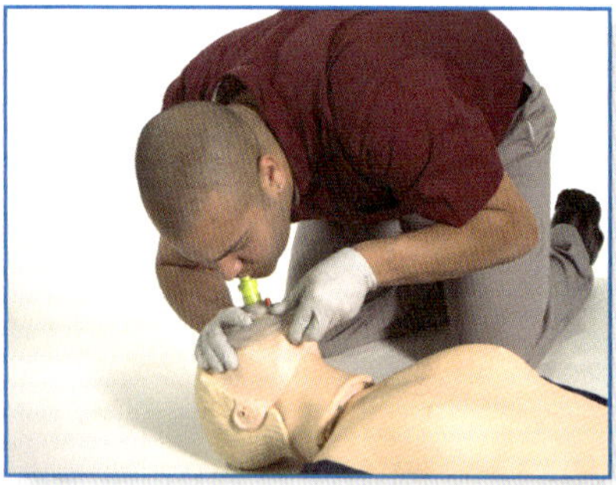

Deliver Breath

- Blow through valve opening to deliver breaths. Each breath is 1 second in length. Give only enough air to create a visible rise of chest, but no more.

Rescue Breaths — CPR Shield

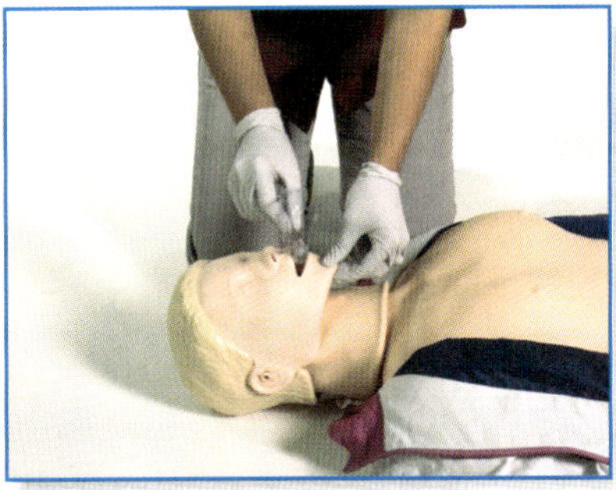

Position Shield

- Place breathing port of shield between teeth and into person's mouth.

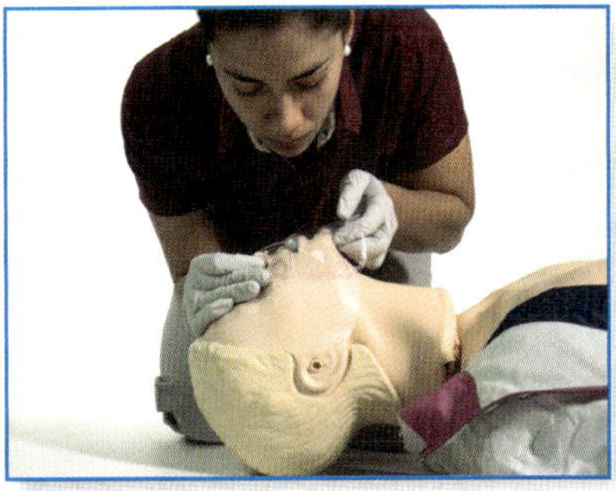

Open Airway

- Place one hand across forehead.
- Hook fingertips of your other hand under bony ridge of chin.
- Tilt head and lift chin to open airway.
- Seal nose by pinching nostrils closed over or under the shield.

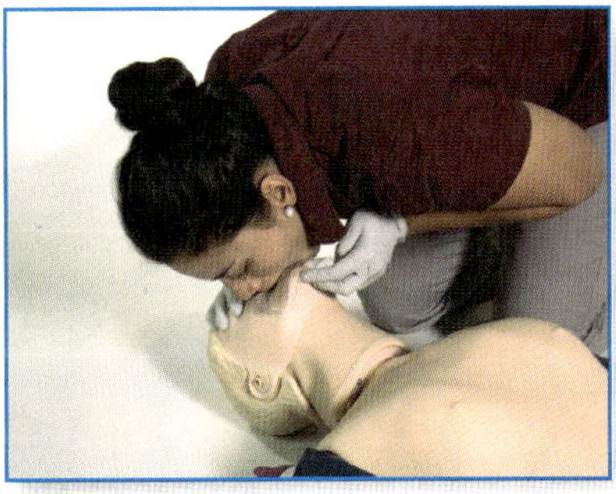

Deliver Breath

- Take a normal breath. Open your mouth wide. Press your mouth on shield around person's mouth to create airtight seal.
- Blow through port to deliver breath. Each breath is 1 second in length. Give only enough air to create a visible rise of chest, but no more.
- Remove your mouth and let person exhale before delivering second rescue breath.

Automated External Defibrillation

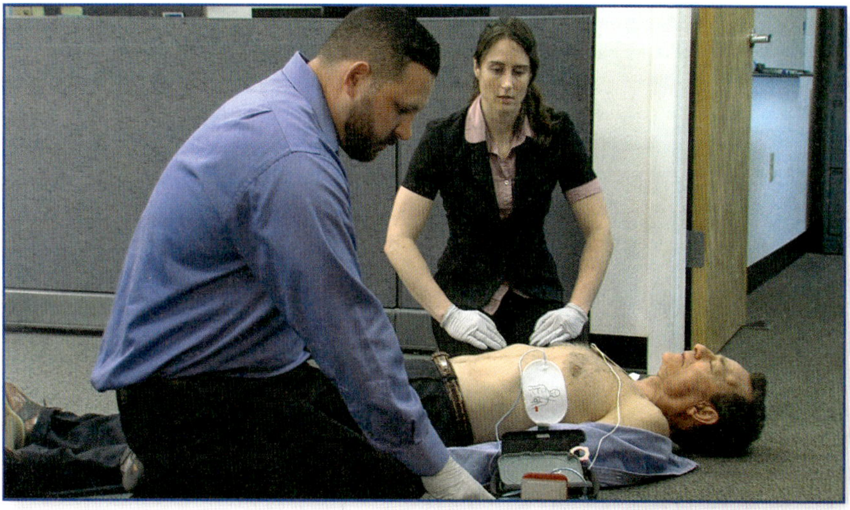

AEDs are designed to be simple to use. Voice, lights, and screen instructions guide a user in operating the device.

AED Operation

There are many different brands of AEDs, but the same basic steps for operation apply to all.

Turn on AED

Opening the lid will turn on the power for some AEDs. With others, simply press the power button. This starts voice instructions and readies the device for use.

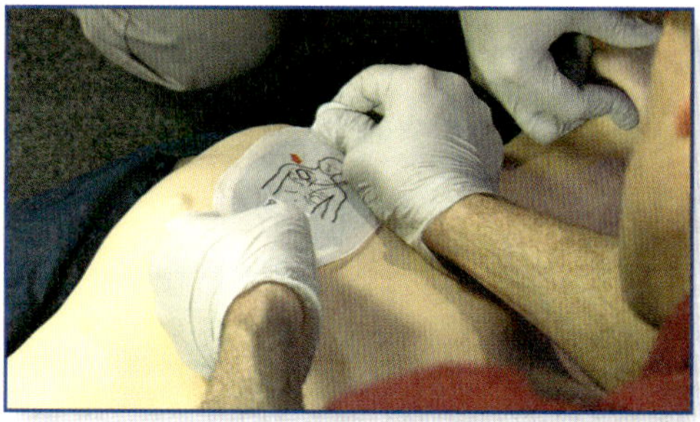

Adhere Defibrillation Pads to Chest

Pads must be applied to a bare chest. If needed, quickly tear away or use scissors to remove all clothing from the torso. For a woman, remove the bra to provide better access for pad placement.

Locate and pull out the defibrillation pads. The pads have pictures on them to show proper placement. Proper placement will assure that the pads are able to direct the electrical shock through the heart. Peel the pads from the backing sheet one at a time and place them as shown in the pictures. Place one pad below the right collarbone, above the nipple, and beside the breastbone. Make sure it adheres well by pressing it flat. Place the other pad lower on the left side, over the ribs, and a few inches below the armpit. Again, press firmly.

Allow AED to Analyze Heart Rhythm

An AED automatically starts analyzing once the pads are in place. Most pads are already connected to the device. Stop CPR. Movement can interrupt the analysis. Be certain that no one is touching the person. If defibrillation is advised, the AED will begin to charge for shock delivery.

Deliver Shock if Directed to by AED

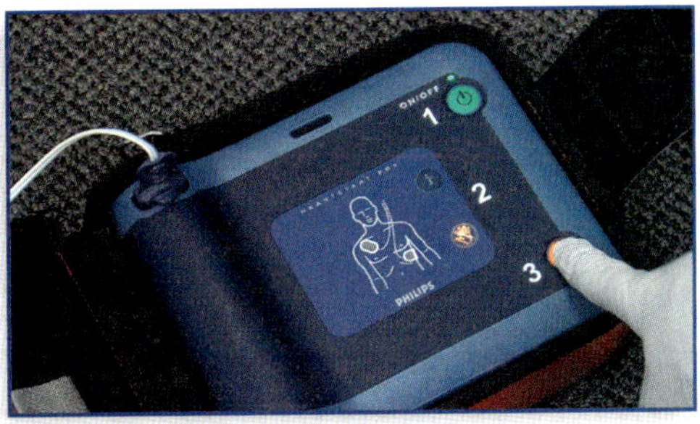

To prevent the accidental shock of a rescuer, quickly look to make sure no one, including you, is in contact with the person before delivering the shock. For most AEDs, a button is pressed to deliver the shock. Once delivered, immediately resume CPR, starting with chest compressions.

AED Troubleshooting & Considerations

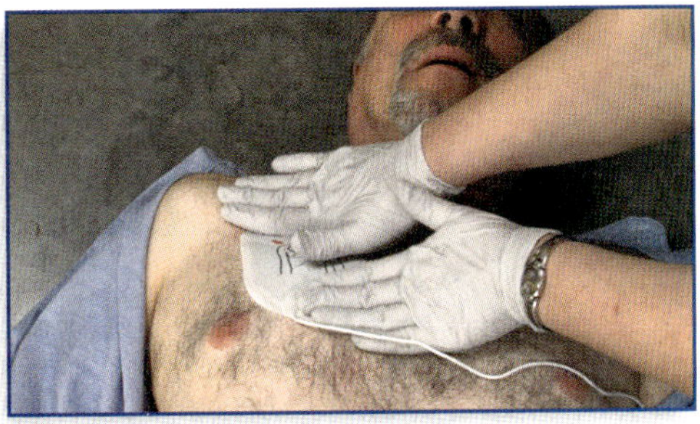

AEDs are also designed to detect problems during use and guide you through corrective actions. If a troubleshooting message occurs at any time, stay calm and follow the AED's voice instructions.

When it becomes necessary to troubleshoot an AED, CPR should be provided, without interruption, until the problem is corrected or another AED becomes available. Pauses of CPR lasting longer than 10 seconds should be avoided.

If the AED indicates a problem with the pads, the pads are not completely adhered to the skin or there is a poor connection to the AED. Press pads firmly, especially in the center, to make sure they are adhering well. Make sure the pads' cable connector is firmly connected to the AED.

If the chest is wet, dry the chest before applying pads. If the chest becomes wet after the pads are applied, remove the pads and dry the chest. Apply a new set of pads, if available.

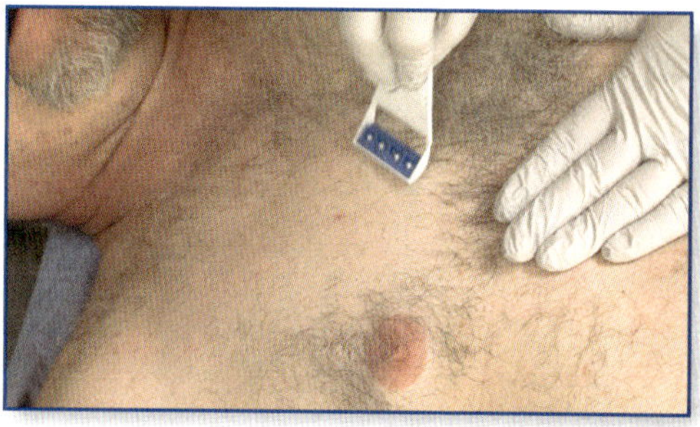

Thick chest hair may prevent the AED pads from adhering to the skin. If chest hair is excessive, quickly shave the hair in the areas where the pads will be placed. If pads were placed over chest hair and do not adhere, pull the pads off quickly and shave the hair. Attach another set of pads, if available. Otherwise, re-apply the original pads.

Another troubleshooting message may indicate that analysis has been interrupted due to movement. Stop all sources of movement, such as chest compressions or rescue breaths.

If a message indicates the need to replace a battery, there may be only enough energy for a limited number of shocks and only a few more minutes of operation. If the AED fails to operate, the depleted battery should be removed and replaced with a new one. If a battery needs replacement during resuscitation, it should be replaced during a CPR interval.

A person should be removed from standing water before using an AED. It is okay to use an AED when a person is lying on a wet surface, such as in the rain or near a swimming pool. An AED should never be immersed in water or have fluids spilled on it.

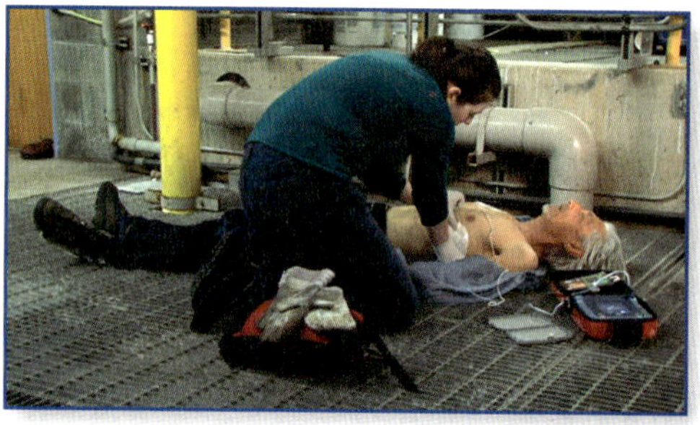

AEDs can also be used safely on metal surfaces, such as gratings or stairwells. Make sure pads do not directly touch any metal surface.

Someone may have a surgically implanted device in the chest, such as a pacemaker or an automated internal defibrillator. A noticeable lump and surgical scar will be visible. If the implanted device is in the way of correct pad placement, place the pads so the edges are at least one inch away from the device.

Defibrillating over medication patches could reduce the effectiveness of the shock. If a medication patch is interfering with placement, use a gloved hand to peel off the patch and wipe away any remaining residue before placing pads.

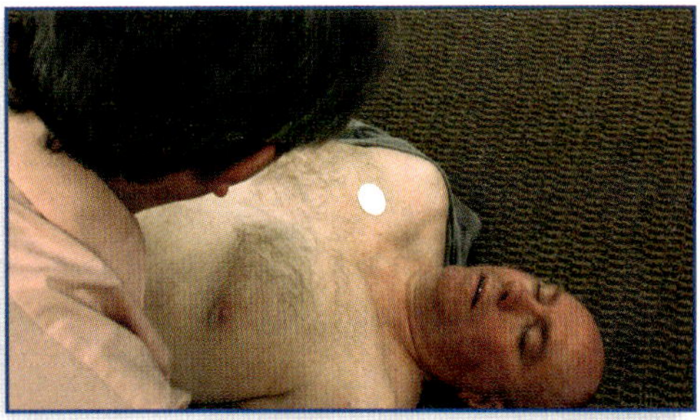

Knowledge Check

You have been asked to respond to a meeting room with an AED. As you enter the room, you see another first aid provider performing chest compressions on a man who is lying on the floor. You kneel next to the man and lay the AED next to his head. What are the 4 basic steps you will take to use the AED on him?

Using an AED

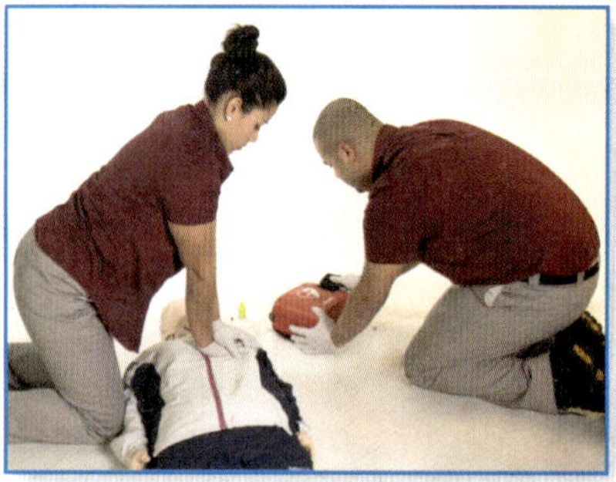

Perform CPR

- If person is unresponsive and not breathing, immediately perform CPR.
- Provide continuous cycles of 30 compressions and 2 rescue breaths.

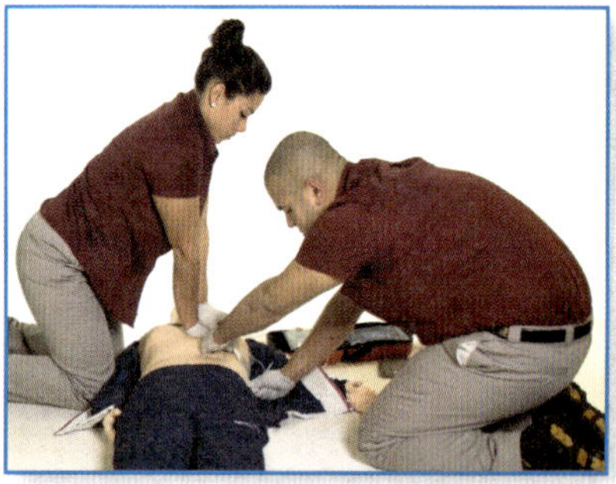

When Available, Attach AED

- Turn on AED and bare person's chest.
- Peel first pad from backing and place below right collarbone, above nipple, and beside breastbone.
- Remove second pad from backing and place on left side, over ribs, and a few inches below armpit.

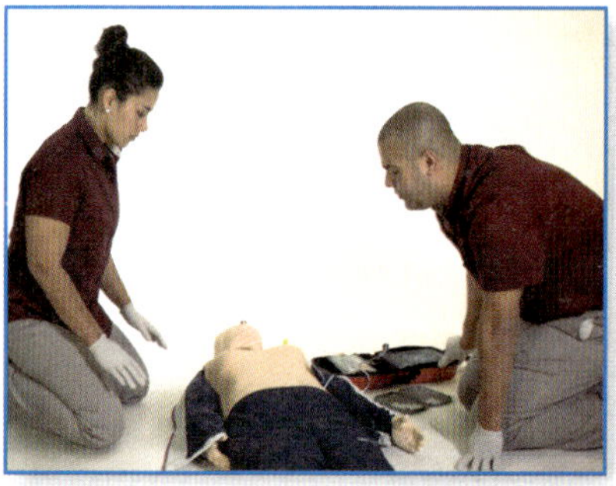

If Indicated, Deliver Shock

- Allow AED to analyze heart. Stop CPR. Do not touch the person.
- If shock is advised, clear everyone and press button to deliver shock.

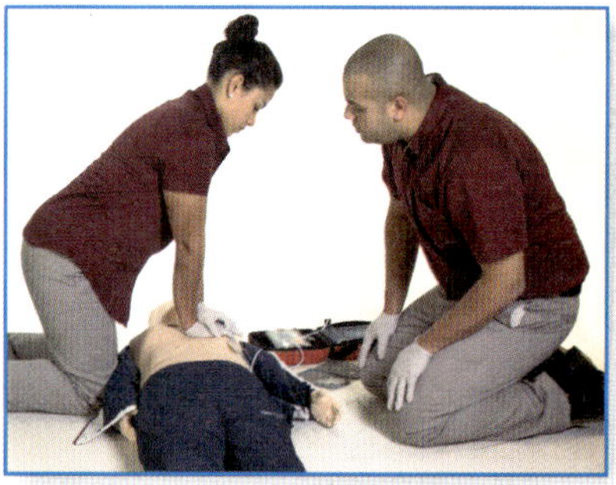

Resume CPR

- Quickly resume CPR with chest compressions. Follow any additional voice instructions from AED.
- Continue until another provider or EMS personnel take over.
- If person responds, stop CPR and place in recovery positon. Leave AED on and attached.

Primary Assessment — Unresponsive Person

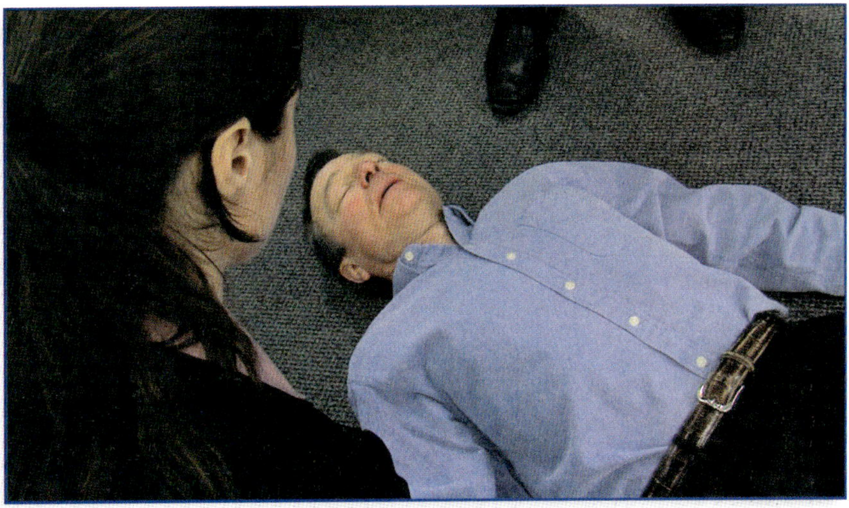

The primary assessment is a simple way to quickly identify if a life-threatening condition is present. It is the initial approach to anyone suspected of being ill or injured.

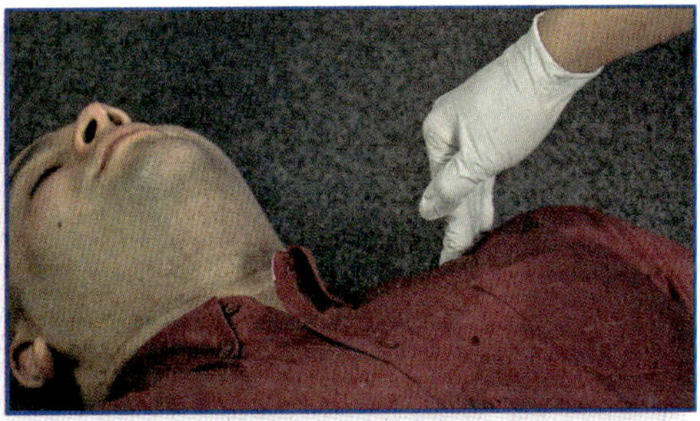

The steps of the primary assessment are always the same:

- If it is safe to provide care, check for responsiveness.
- If unresponsive, activate EMS and get an AED, if one is available.
- Check for normal breathing.
- If normal breathing is found, place an uninjured person in a recovery position.
- If the person is not breathing or only gasping, perform CPR.

If you determine a person is unresponsive, send a bystander to activate EMS and get an AED. If you are alone, do this yourself and quickly return to the person.

If you have a mobile phone, use it to activate EMS. The speaker function will allow you to follow instructions from an EMS dispatcher while providing care.

To check for normal breathing, quickly look at the face and chest. Take no longer than 10 seconds. Normal breathing is effortless, quiet, and regular. If you are unsure, assume breathing is not normal.

Weak, irregular gasping, snorting, or gurgling sounds can occur early in cardiac arrest. These actions provide no usable oxygen. This is not normal breathing.

If the person is not breathing, or only gasping, perform CPR, beginning with compressions.

When an unresponsive person is breathing normally, and uninjured, place him or her in a side-lying recovery position to help protect the airway.

Recovery Position

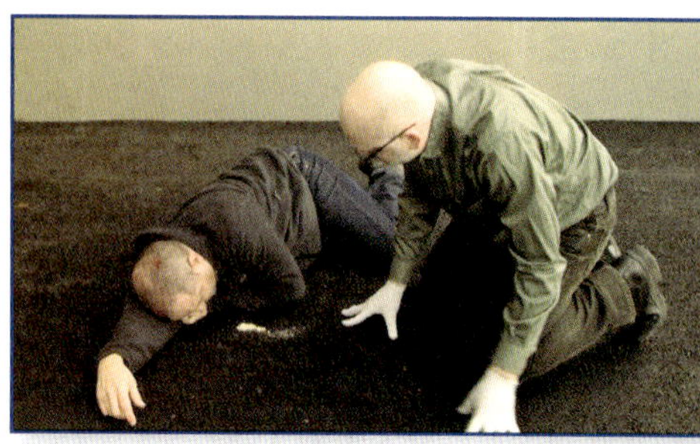

The recovery position helps protect the airway by using gravity to drain fluids from the mouth and keep the tongue from blocking the airway.

Frequently assess the breathing of anyone placed in the recovery position. The person's condition could quickly become worse and require additional care.

Knowledge Check

A fellow employee collapses near you during a staff meeting. As a trained first aid provider, you move to help. You kneel next to him, squeeze his shoulder, and loudly ask, "Are you all right?" He is unresponsive, so you direct other employees to activate EMS and get the company's AED. You look closely at the face and chest for breathing; he makes a brief gasping snort, but then remains still. What do you do next?

Primary Assessment — Unresponsive Person

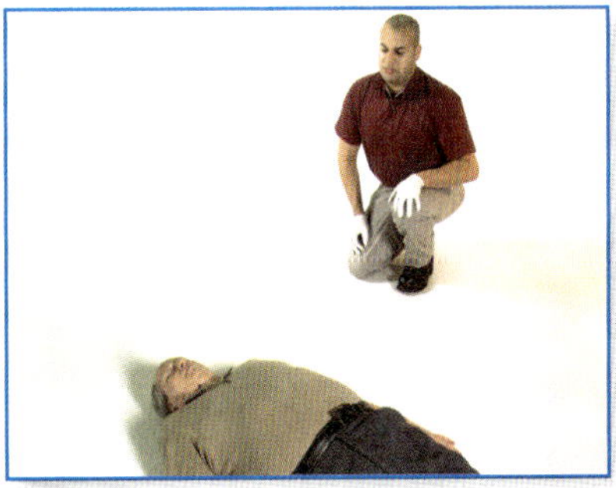

Assess Scene

- Pause and assess scene for safety.
- If unsafe, or if it becomes unsafe at any time, GET OUT!

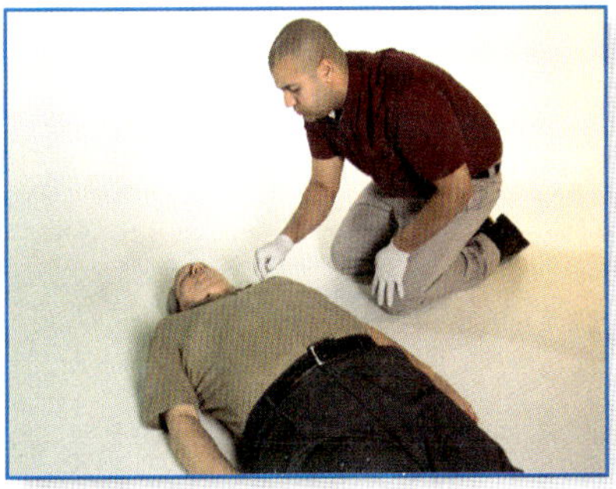

Check for Response

- Tap or squeeze shoulder and ask loudly, "Are you all right?"
- If unresponsive, have someone activate EMS and get an AED.

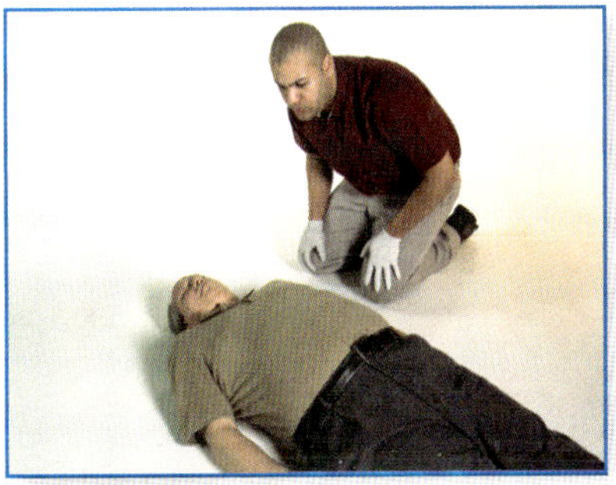

Look for Normal Breathing

- Position person face-up on a firm, flat surface.
- Look at face and chest for normal breathing. Take no longer than 10 seconds. If unsure, assume breathing is not normal.
- Weak, irregular gasping, snorting, or gurgling is not normal breathing.

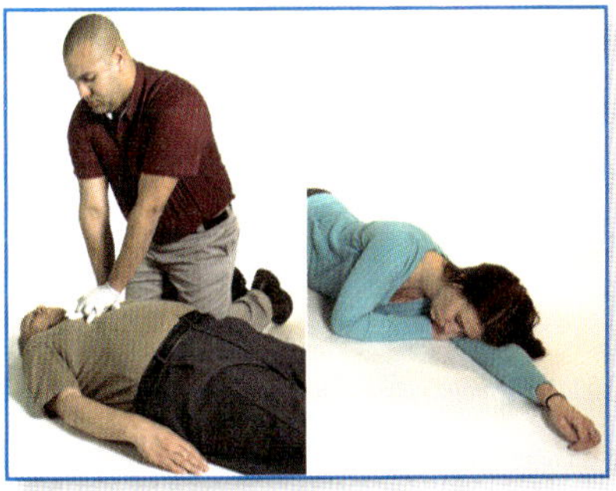

Provide Indicated Care

- If person is not breathing, or only gasping, perform CPR, beginning with compressions.
- If normal breathing is found, place an uninjured person in recovery position.

Recovery Position

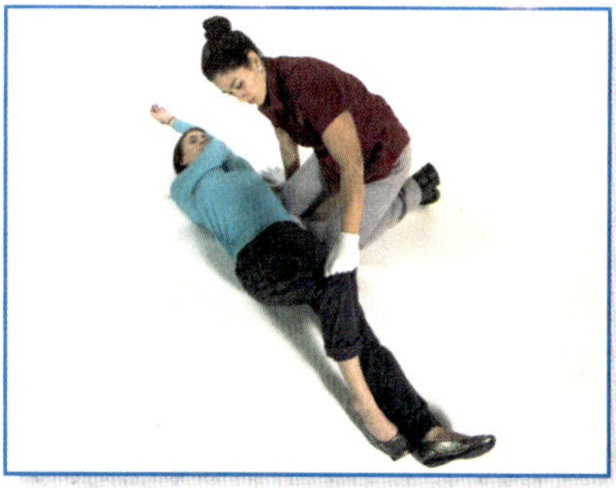

Prepare

- Place arm nearest you up alongside head.
- Bring far arm across chest and place back of hand against cheek.
- Grasp far leg just above knee and pull it up so the foot is flat on ground.

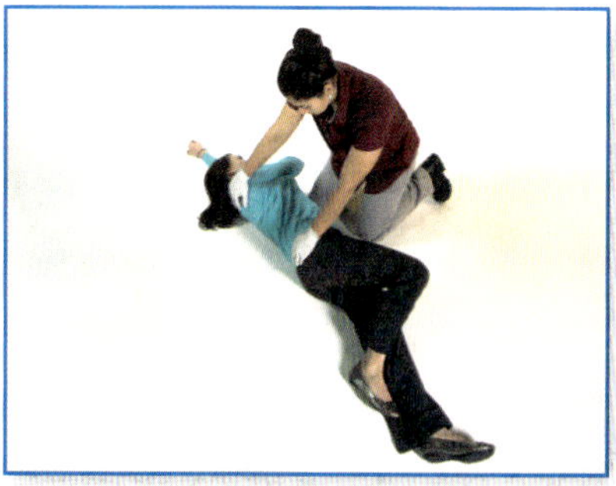

Roll

- Grasping shoulder and hip, roll person toward you in a single motion, keeping head, shoulders, and body from twisting.
- Roll far enough for face to be angled toward ground.

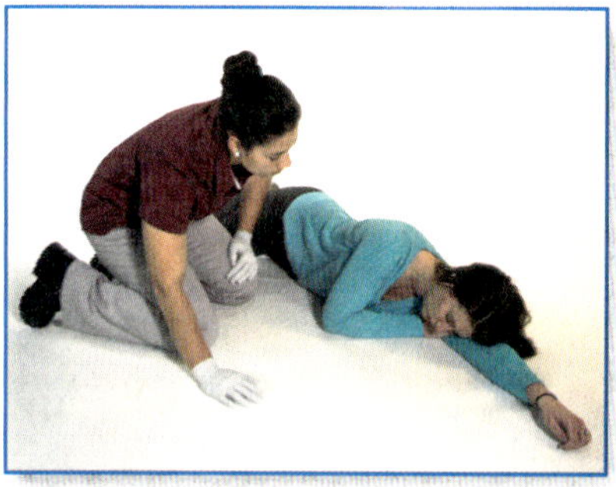

Stabilize

- Position elbow and legs to stabilize head and body. Ensure there is no pressure on chest that restricts breathing.
- Make sure head ends up resting on extended arm and head, neck, and body are aligned.
- If person has been seriously injured, do not move unless fluids are in airway, or you need to leave to get help.

Caring for Cardiac Arrest

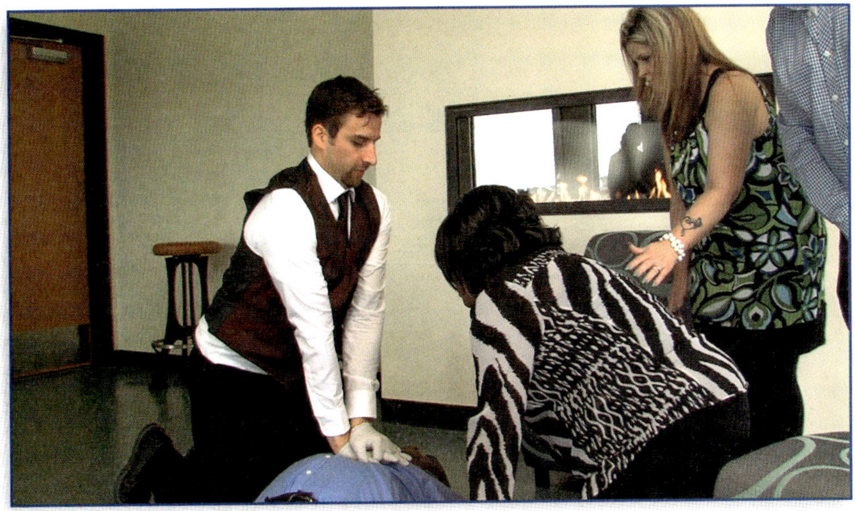

Immediate, high-quality CPR and defibrillation with an AED from a bystander can double or even triple the chance of surviving sudden cardiac arrest.

Before anything else, pause and assess the scene for hazards. If the situation is dangerous to you, do not approach.

If it is safe, quickly assess for responsiveness. If unresponsive, send someone to activate EMS and get an AED.

Check for normal breathing. Do not be fooled by gasping actions. If not breathing, or only gasping, begin compressions at 100 to 120 times per minute. Remember that quality matters. Push hard and push fast. Do not lean on the chest.

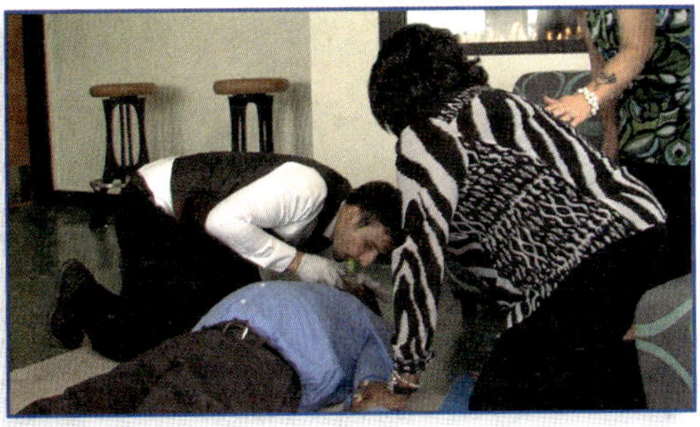

After 30 compressions, give 2 rescue breaths. Establish an airway first and give only enough air to see the chest rise but no more. Do this quickly, in less than 10 seconds.

Return to compressions and perform ongoing CPR cycles of 30 compressions and 2 rescue breaths. Compress hard and fast, and allow the chest to fully recoil to its normal position after each compression.

Use the AED immediately when it arrives. If another person is available to operate the AED, do not stop CPR. Continue compressions as best you can until the AED is ready to analyze the heart rhythm.

Turn on the AED and adhere the defibrillation pads to the bare chest. Allow the AED to analyze the heart. If a shock is advised, make sure you are not touching the person before delivering the shock.

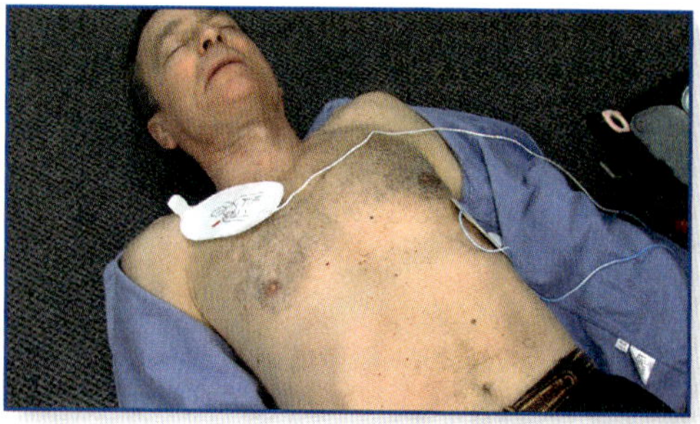

Immediately after a shock is delivered, resume CPR starting with compressions. Voice instructions and additional analysis by the AED will guide you through further care. Don't stop until the person shows signs of life, another provider or EMS personnel take over, or you are too exhausted to continue.

If a person clearly responds, stop CPR and place the person in the recovery position. Leave the AED on and attached in case cardiac arrest returns.

If a shock is not indicated by the AED, immediately resume CPR. Continue to follow the AED's instructions.

Blood pressure is created and maintained with ongoing compressions. When compressions stop, pressure is quickly lost and has to be built up again. Avoid interruptions to maintain high-quality CPR.

Performing effective chest compressions is tiring. When others can help, take turns performing CPR. Quickly switch compressors every few minutes. When possible, do this during the automatic AED analysis that occurs every 2 minutes.

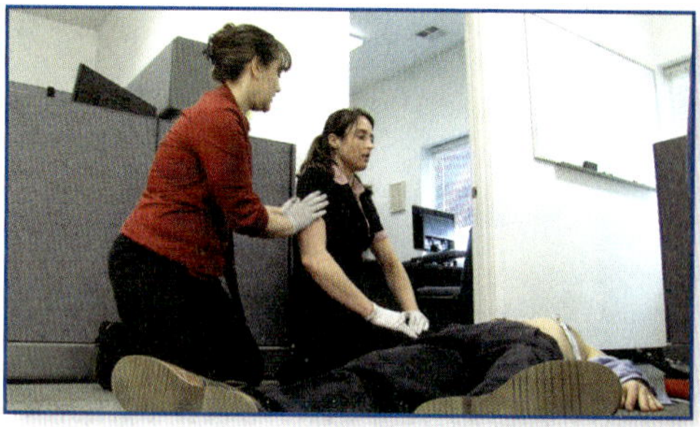

Do the best you can. A person without breathing or circulation will not survive without help. Nothing you can do can make the outcome worse.

Compression-only CPR is an approach that is being widely promoted to people who are not trained in CPR.

Simple instructions in compression-only CPR can be shared in many different ways, including social media and as public service announcements. EMS dispatchers can also provide compression-only instructions during an emergency call.

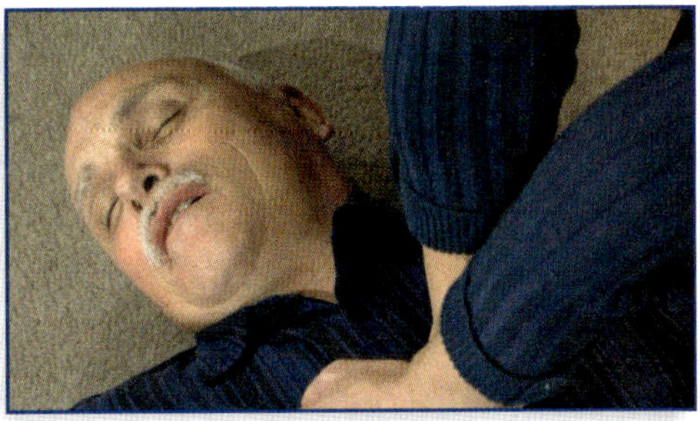

However, compression-only CPR is a limited approach. At some point, rescue breaths are essential for all cardiac arrests, especially those involving an airway or breathing problem, or those involving children.

As a trained provider, perform both compressions and breaths during CPR. If you are unable or unwilling to perform rescue breaths, you should provide high-quality, uninterrupted compressions at a minimum.

Special CPR Situations

- **Fluids in Airway** — Roll person on side to quickly drain fluids. Roll without twisting, like a log. Remove any material still in mouth with a gloved finger.
- **Cold Environments** — Handle cold people gently to prevent cardiac arrest. If body is solid, do not start CPR.
- **Drowning** — As quickly and safely as possible, get person onto solid ground. Expect vomiting. Do not attempt to expel water using abdominal thrusts.
- **Serious Injury** — Someone in cardiac arrest due to injury is unlikely to survive. If it is clear injury has caused arrest, do not start CPR.
- **Electric Shock/Lightning** — Approach only if it is safe. Electric shock can cause ventricular fibrillation. When safe, perform CPR and use an AED.
- **Neck Breather** — Provide rescue breaths through surgical opening, or stoma, in neck using CPR mask or shield.

Knowledge Check

You have responded to a store customer who collapsed. Your primary assessment indicated she was in cardiac arrest and you have started CPR. Another employee has gone to activate EMS and get an AED. Describe the basic details for performing CPR and using an AED in this situation.

Caring for Cardiac Arrest

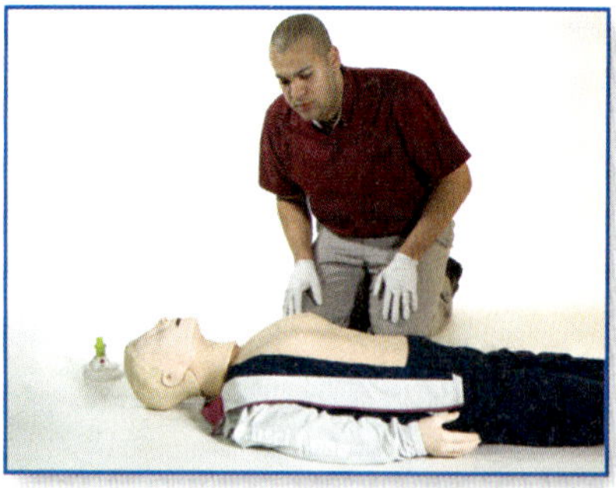

Assess Person

- If safe, tap or squeeze shoulder. Ask loudly, "Are you all right?"
  No response!
- Have someone activate EMS and get an AED.
- Check face and chest for normal breathing.
  Normal breathing absent!

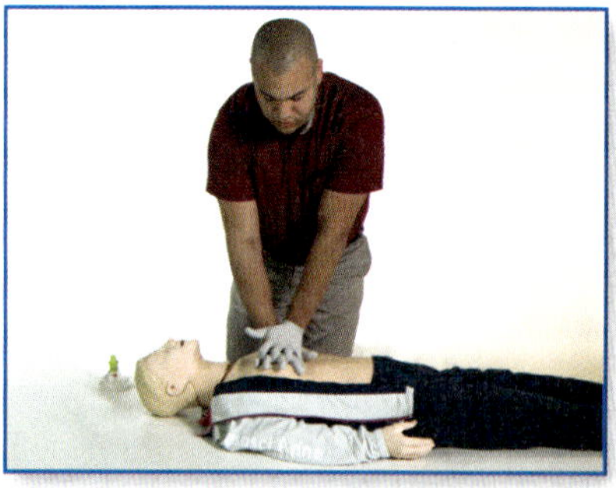

Give 30 Compressions

- Place heel of one hand on center of chest. Place heel of other hand on top of first.
- Bring body up and over chest, using upper body weight to push down hard, at least 2 inches.
- Push fast, at a rate of 100–120 times per minute. Allow chest to fully recoil.

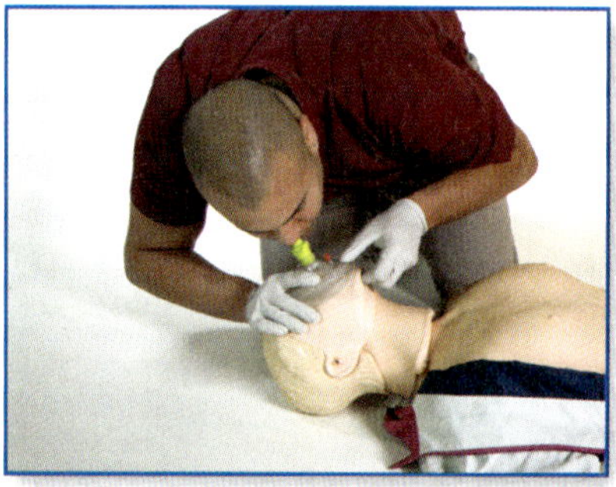

Give 2 Rescue Breaths

- Using a barrier device, tilt head, lift chin to open airway.
- Make chest visibly rise with each breath, but no more.
- Take a fresh breath between rescue breaths. Give breaths in less than 10 seconds
- Provide continuous cycles of 30 compressions and 2 rescue breaths.

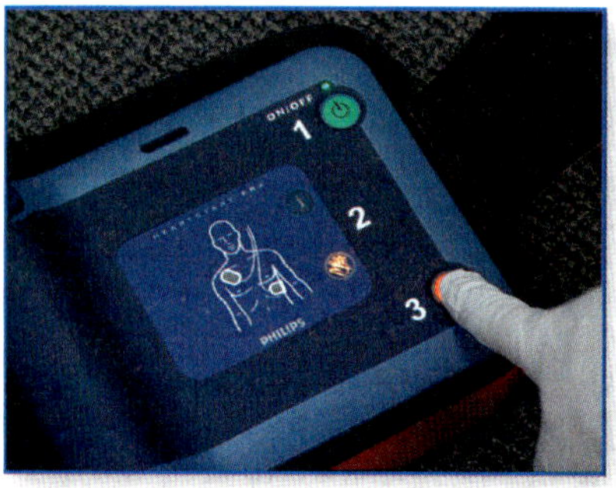

Use an AED

- If AED becomes available, stop CPR and use it immediately. Turn AED on and follow its voice instructions.
- Deliver a shock if indicated by AED. Immediately resume CPR after a shock is delivered or no shock is advised.
- Continue until another provider or EMS personnel take over, the person shows signs of life, or you are too exhausted to continue.

Multiple Provider Approach to CPR

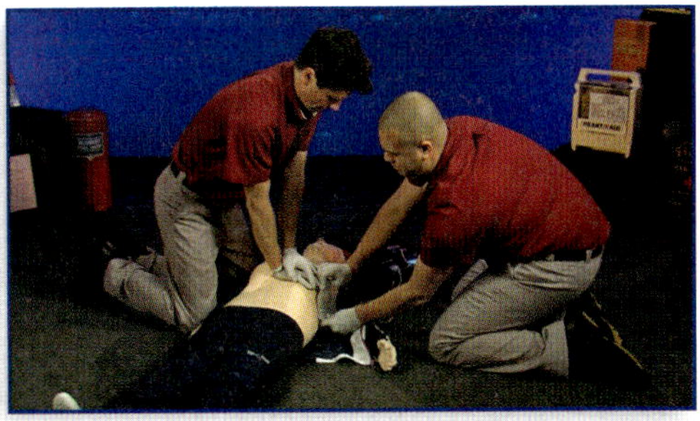

Commonly more than one trained provider is available to help when cardiac arrest occurs. Providers can work together to improve performance and reduce interruptions.

CPR is tiring, and switching providers about every 2 minutes helps to maintain CPR quality. Communicate about switches ahead of time. Coordinate your actions to switch smoothly and minimize interruption time.

Prior to AED Arrival

Switch at the end of a CPR cycle while the person who is going to move out is giving rescue breaths. The new provider can get into position to start compressions. When rescue breaths are completed, immediately resume compressions.

When an AED Arrives

If another person is available to operate the AED, do not stop CPR. Continue compressions as best you can until the AED is ready to analyze the heart rhythm.

After an AED is Attached

Switch when the AED analyzes the heart. This occurs about every 2 minutes. The new CPR provider gets into position to perform compressions and the new AED provider gets in place to operate the AED. After a shock is delivered or if no shock is indicated, immediately start compressions.

When 2 providers are present, simply take turns doing CPR. Rotate extra providers in if more than 2 providers are present.

Knowledge Check

As a trained first aid provider, you respond to a situation in which CPR is already being performed for an employee who has collapsed. An AED is coming but has not yet arrived. The CPR provider looks exhausted. How would you smoothly integrate yourself to take over doing the CPR?

Multiple Provider Approach to CPR

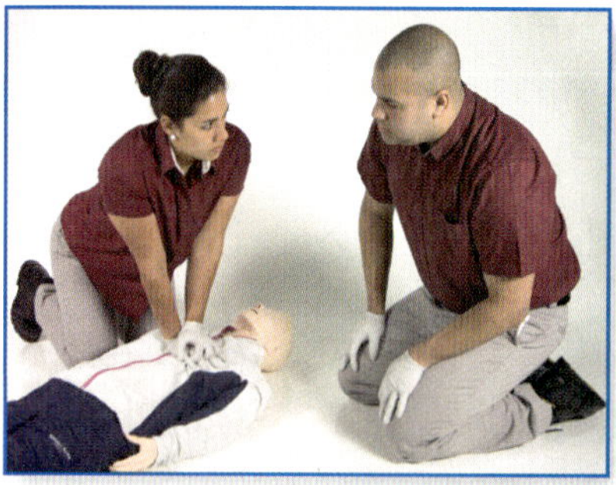

Consider a Switch

- CPR is tiring. When available, switch CPR providers about every 2 minutes.
- Clearly communicate switches ahead of time so everyone understands.

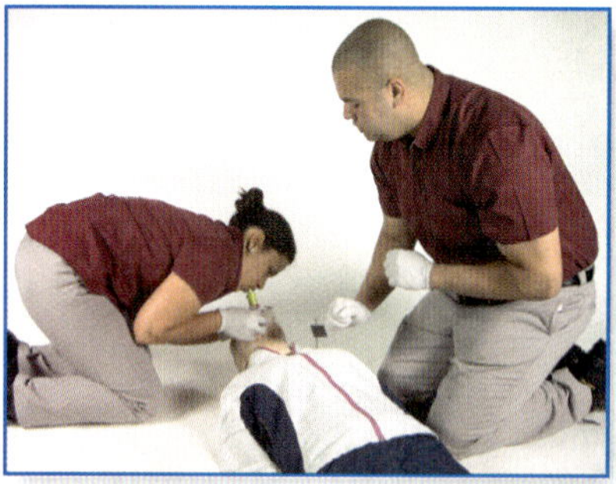

Prior to the Arrival of an AED

- Incoming CPR provider moves into place while outgoing provider is giving rescue breaths.
- New CPR provider immediately begins compressions when rescue breaths are completed.

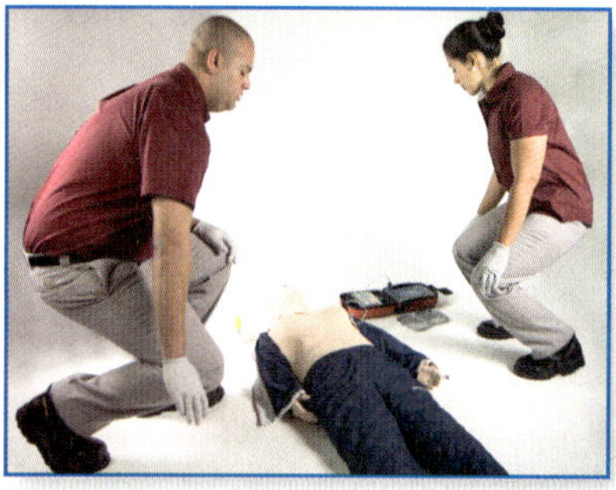

When an AED Is Attached

- Switch roles when AED analyzes heart. This occurs about every 2 minutes.
- Immediately begin compressions after a shock is delivered or when AED advises no shock is indicated.

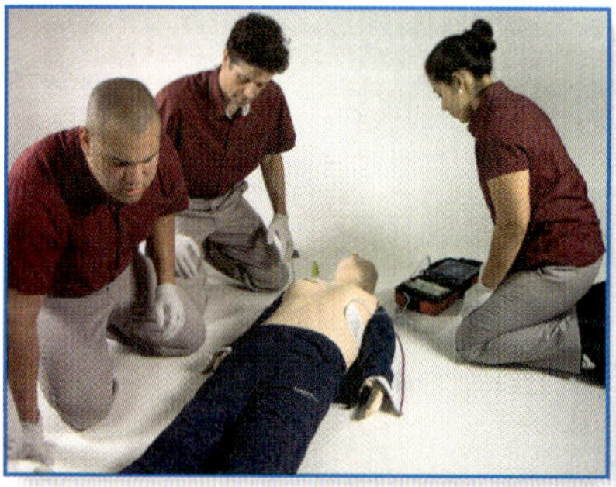

More than 2 Providers

- Rotate extra providers in if more than 2 providers are present.

Choking

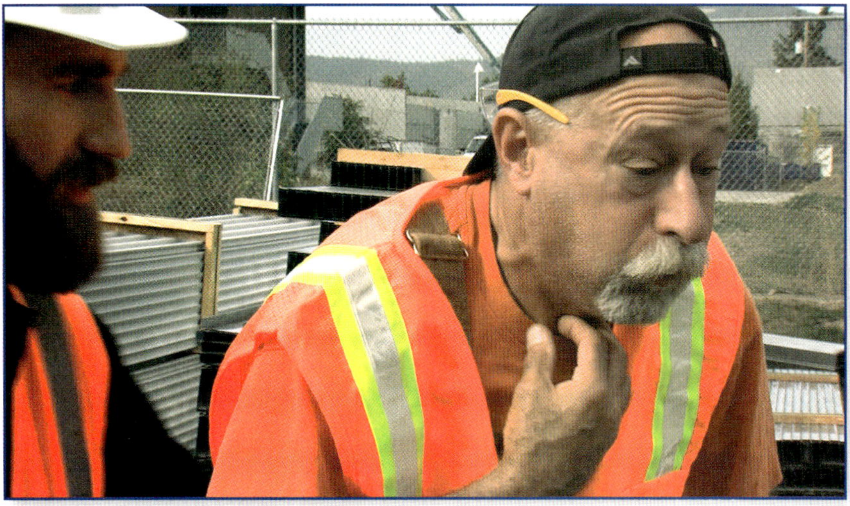

Choking can occur when a solid object, such as a piece of food, or a small object, enters a narrowed part of the airway and becomes stuck. On inhalation, the object can be drawn tighter into the airway and block air from entering the lungs.

A forceful thrust beneath the ribs and up into the diaphragm can pressurize the air in the chest and pop an obstruction out of the airway. Compression of the chest over the breastbone can also create enough pressure to expel an object.

Mild Obstruction

To provide the appropriate care, you must first be able to recognize the difference between a mild blockage and a severe blockage.

With a mild blockage, a person can speak, cough, or gag. This type of blockage is typically cleared naturally through forceful coughing. Allow someone with a mild blockage to try and resolve the problem on his or her own. Stay close and be ready to take action if things worsen.

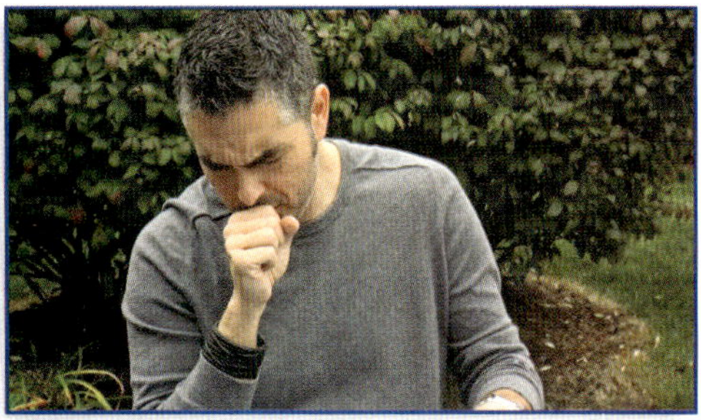

Severe Obstruction

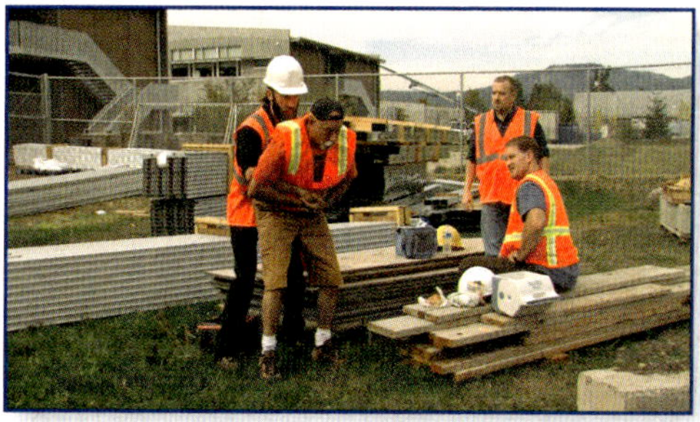

When a severe blockage occurs, a person cannot take in enough air to dislodge the object. Signs of severe obstruction include very little or no air exchange, lack of sound, and the inability to speak or cough forcefully. The person may hold his or her hands to the throat while attempting to clear the obstruction.

A person without any air exchange requires your help to survive.

PREGNANT OR OBESE

When someone is clearly pregnant or obese, use chest thrusts instead of abdominal thrusts.

SELF-CARE

If you are choking and alone, try pressing your abdomen quickly against a rigid surface, such as falling onto the back of a chair. If one is not available, attempt abdominal thrusts on yourself.

Knowledge Check

You are in the company cafeteria eating lunch with a coworker. He is laughing at something you said when he suddenly stops, grasps his throat with his hands, and stands up quickly. He clearly looks distressed, so you stand up next to him and ask, “Are you choking?” He is unable to answer you and completely silent. You decide to perform abdominal thrusts. Describe how to perform them.

Choking

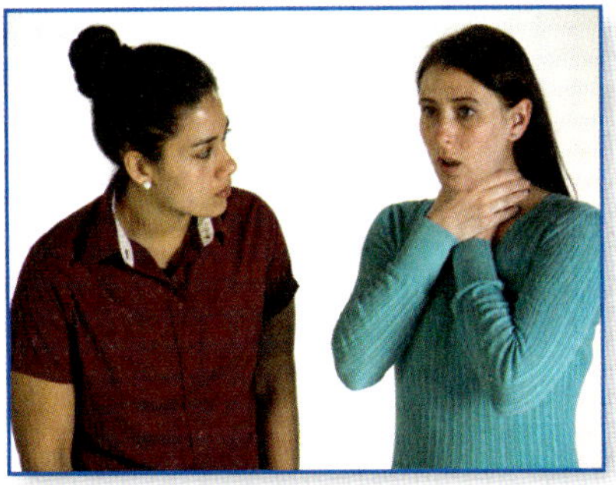

Assess Person

- Ask, "Are you choking?"
- If person nods yes, or is unable to speak or cough, act quickly.
- If available, have a bystander activate EMS.

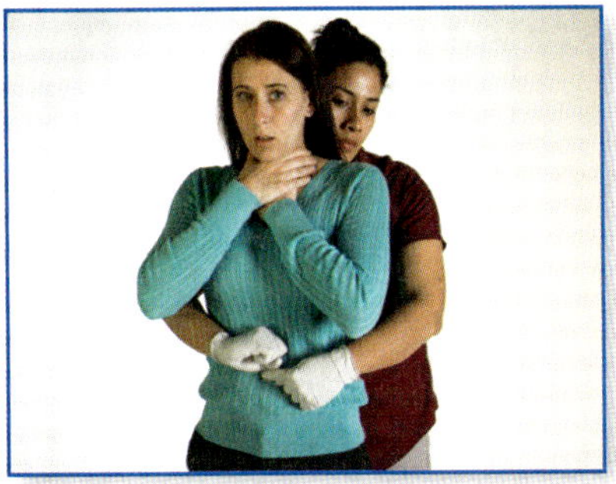

Position Yourself

- Stand behind person. Reach around and locate navel.
- Make a fist with other hand and place thumb side against abdomen, just above navel and below ribs.
- Grasp fist with other hand.

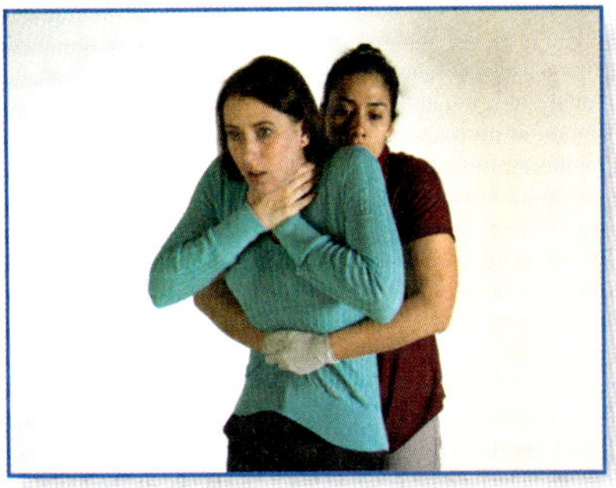

Give Thrusts

- Quickly thrust inward and upward into abdomen.
- Repeat. Each thrust needs to be given with intent of expelling object.
- Continue until person can breathe normally.

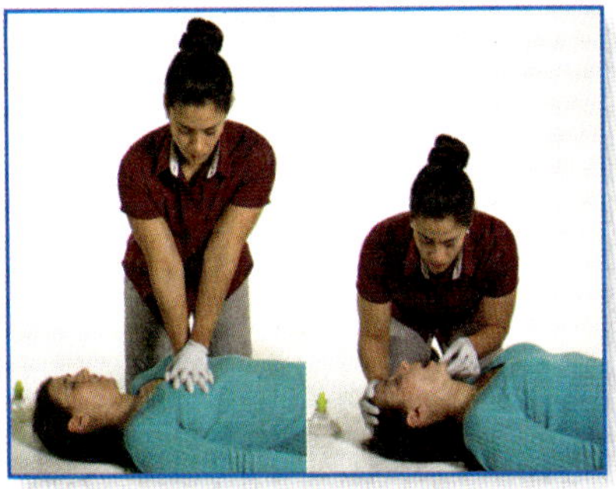

If Person Becomes Unresponsive

- Carefully lower person to ground.
- If not already done, activate EMS and get an AED, if one is available.
- Begin CPR, starting with compressions.
- Look in mouth for an object before giving rescue breaths. Remove any object seen.
- Continue CPR until person shows obvious signs of life, or another provider or EMS personnel take over.

Primary Assessment — Responsive Person

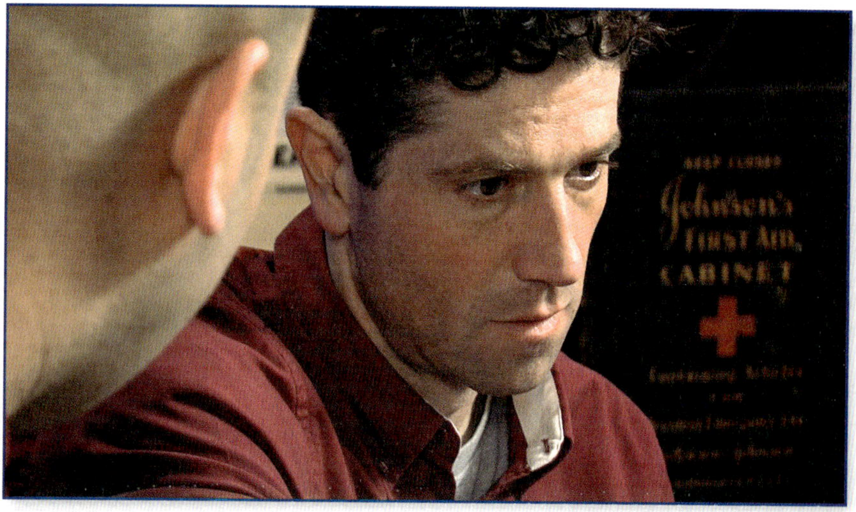

The primary assessment remains the same for a responsive person as it is for an unresponsive person.

Look for any immediately life-threatening problems. Introduce yourself and see if there is any diminished level of responsiveness, altered mental status, or difficulty in breathing. Briefly scan the body for serious bleeding. If found, control it immediately.

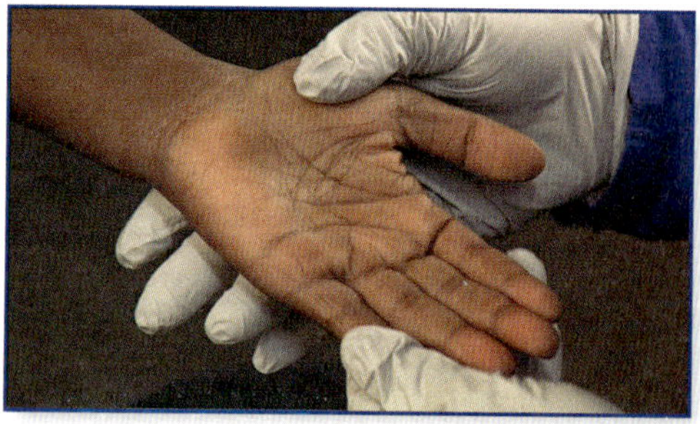

Look for obvious signs of shock. Check the face for tissue color. Tissue color indicates the amount of blood circulating below the skin:

- Normal tissue color is light pink.
- Paleness indicates blood loss or shock.
- A bluish color indicates a lack of oxygen.

Depending on skin tone, it may be easier to look at tissue color in the palms of hands, fingernails, or inside the lip.

Check skin temperature by touching the forehead with your bare wrist:

- Normal skin feels warm and dry.
- Cool, wet skin can be an indication of shock.

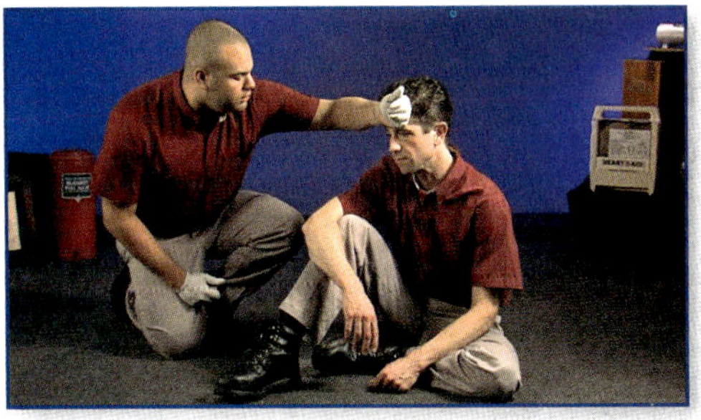

If a life-threatening medical condition is found or suspected, immediately activate EMS and provide any indicated care.

Ongoing Assessment

Emergencies are dynamic events that can change at any time. Reassessment is the ongoing observation of an ill or injured person to monitor his or her condition and the effectiveness of first aid.

Make sure the situation remains safe for you to be there. Watch for changes in a person's level of responsiveness. Ensure the airway is open and clear and that the person is breathing normally. Reassess to ensure external bleeding is controlled. Look for changes in the person's tissue color or skin temperature. Check at regular intervals until another provider or EMS personnel take over.

Knowledge Check

You are stacking shelves in the home goods area of the store where you work when you hear a loud crash and the sound of glass shattering. As a trained first aid provider, you cautiously move to see what happened. A frightened-looking customer is sitting on the floor next to a display that has collapsed. She is surrounded by broken glass. You carefully get to her and let her know you are trained and can help. She appears aware of what happened and is breathing normally. You scan the floor around her and see a growing pool of blood behind her. The back of her blouse is soaked with blood. What do you do next?

Primary Assessment — Responsive Person

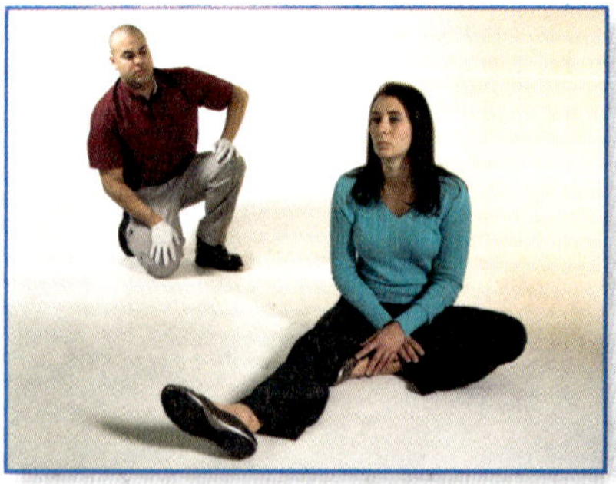

Assess Scene

- Pause and assess scene for safety.
- If unsafe, or if it becomes unsafe at any time, GET OUT!

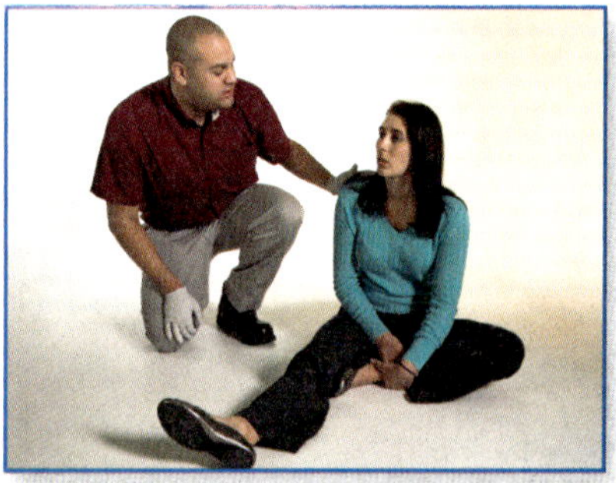

Introduce Yourself

- Tell person you are first aid trained and ask if you can help.
- Check for diminished level of responsiveness or altered mental status.
- Assess for any breathing difficulty.

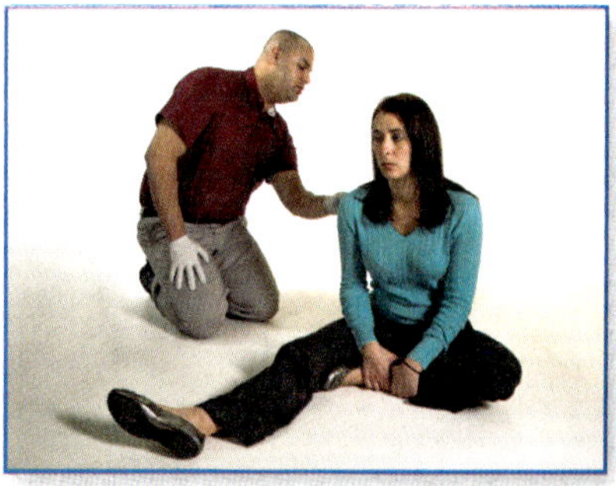

Check for Bleeding

- Scan body for heavy bleeding. If found, control it immediately.

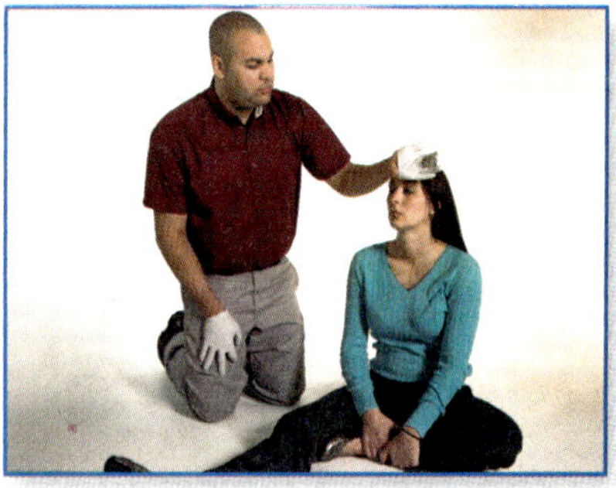

Check Tissue Color and Temperature

- Look at face to check tissue color. Depending on skin tone, it may be easier to check tissue color on the palms, fingernails, or inside the lip.
- Touch person's forehead with your bare wrist to assess body temperature.
- Activate EMS and provide any care when a life-threatening condition is found or suspected.

Secondary Assessment

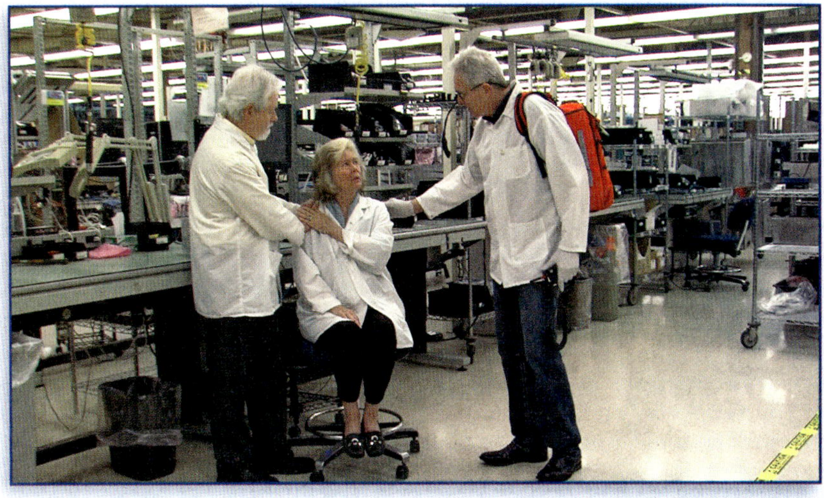

When a primary assessment indicates no life-threatening problems, consider performing a secondary assessment.

A secondary assessment is an organized approach to gather more information about an ill or injured person. It is the same regardless of the situation.

If you find or begin to suspect a life-threatening problem is occurring while performing a secondary assessment, stop, quickly activate EMS, and provide the necessary care.

Begin by trying to identify what happened. Determine if the person has a primary, or chief, complaint.

- If the person cannot answer, ask bystanders.
- Consider hidden injuries if any significant force impacted the body.
- If at any time you suspect an injury to the head, neck, or back, immediately instruct the person to remain still.
- Look around. Clues, such as the presence of medications or containers, may also help identify what happened.
- Check if the person has a medical alert bracelet or necklace identifying an underlying medical condition.

Physically assess the person. Briefly evaluate the body moving from head to toe. Look and feel for signs of illness and injury.

The DOTS mnemonic device can help you remember what to look for during a physical assessment:

- Deformities: Unusual body presentation, differences from other side
- Open injuries: Bleeding injuries
- Tenderness: Painful areas, especially when touched
- Swelling: Swollen and discolored body areas

If covered, remove or cut away clothing to get a better look at an injured or painful body part.

Ask questions to gather more information. Use the mnemonic device SAMPLE to help you remember what to ask about:

- Signs and symptoms: Things the person is feeling, such as pain, nausea, dizziness; anything related to the situation
- Allergies: Things the person may be allergic to
- Medications: Medications the person has been prescribed or is taking
- Past medical problems: Medical problems that may be related to what is going on
- Last oral intake: When and what the person last ate or drank
- Events leading to the problem: What the person was doing just prior to the problem occurring

If a secondary assessment reveals any specific problems, provide the indicated care. If you are unsure or concerned about what is going on, activate EMS.

Prioritization of Care

When there are multiple people affected in an emergency, treat the most seriously ill or injured first. Bypass those with minor problems or even ask them for their help. Leave anyone who is obviously dead alone. Focus first on those who have immediate life threatening problems, and then move on to those who still need intervention.

Knowledge Check

A visitor has tripped on a short staircase at the government building where you work. As a trained first aid provider, you have been asked to respond. You find him seated on a bench near the stairs with another employee talking to him. A quick primary assessment shows there are no immediate life-threats. He describes tripping on a step and falling down onto his hands and knees. What are the two techniques you will use to gather more information?

Secondary Assessment

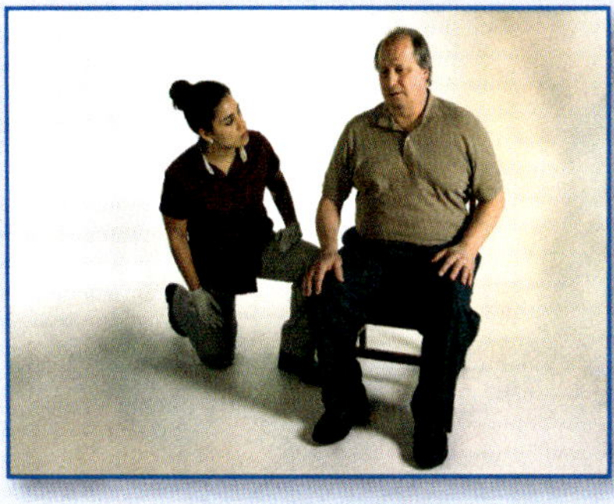

Determine Chief Complaint

- Ask what happened. If person cannot answer, ask bystanders.
- Look for medical alert bracelet or necklace.
- Consider if any mechanism or significant force impacted the body.

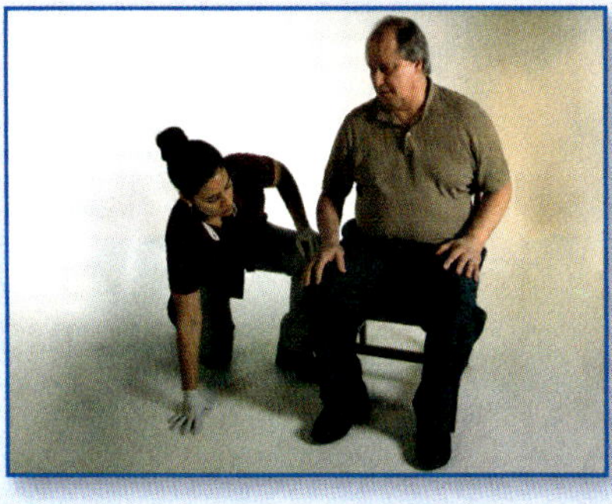

Look at Person

- Quickly scan the body from head to toe.
- Look and feel for signs of illness and injury (**DOTS**):
  - **D**eformities
  - **O**pen injuries
  - **T**enderness
  - **S**welling

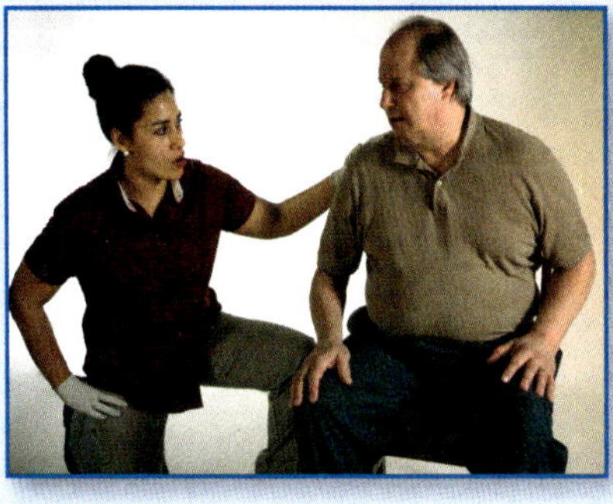

Ask Questions

- Gather more information related to what is going on (**SAMPLE**):
  - **S**ymptoms?
  - **A**llergies?
  - **M**edications?
  - **P**ast medical history?
  - **L**ast oral intake?
  - **E**vents leading up?
- Activate EMS anytime a serious condition is found or suspected.

Control of Bleeding

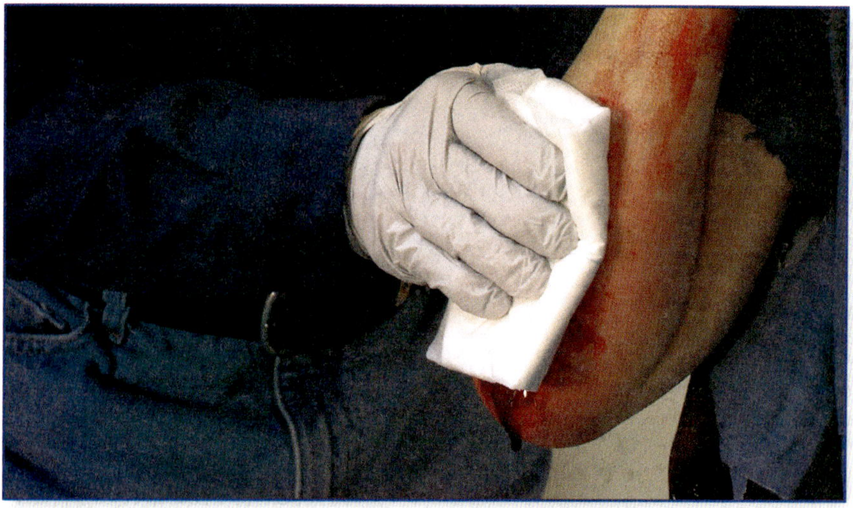

Sudden injuries occur quickly, often from traumatic events, and may become life threatening.

Bleeding occurs when blood vessels, found throughout the body, are damaged. Heavy bleeding is likely if a large blood vessel is involved.

Arterial bleeding is bright red and will often spurt from a wound. It can be difficult to control due to the pressure created by the heart's contractions. If blood is dark red and flowing steadily, it is likely coming from a damaged vein.

Clot-forming fibers naturally collect at a wound site to try to stop bleeding, but heavy bleeding can overwhelm this and prevent clotting from occurring. Bleeding reduces the amount of oxygen that can be delivered to the body. If heavy or uncontrolled, bleeding can quickly become life threatening.

Pressure applied directly to a bleeding site until bleeding stops is the standard method for controlling external bleeding. Activate EMS immediately for any heavy bleeding.

Bleeding exposes you, the provider, to potentially infectious body fluids. Always use disposable gloves as a barrier to protect both you and the injured person. When gloves are not available, an improvised barrier, such as a plastic bag, can be used.

Tourniquets

If direct pressure is unable to control bleeding on a limb, use a tourniquet. Tourniquets utilize a simple binding method around a limb to stop blood flow.

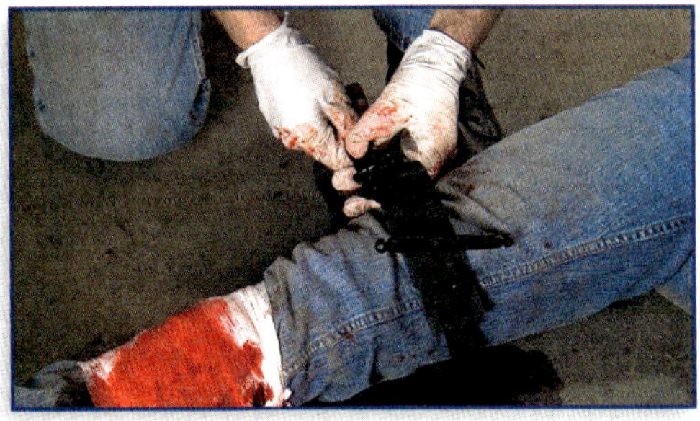

Commercially made tourniquets are ready and easier to use than improvised ones. A compressing band is snugly placed around a limb a few inches above the open injury. A solid handle, connected to the band, is twisted to tighten the band evenly around the limb until bleeding stops. The handle is secured in place to maintain the constriction.

Improvised tourniquets, using the same concept, can be created with nearby materials such as triangular bandages and something solid to twist with.

A tourniquet can also be considered as a primary step to control severe limb bleeding when it is clear direct pressure cannot be used, such as in a mass casualty event, for a person with large or multiple injuries, in a dangerous environment, or for an inaccessible wound.

Training in the application of a tourniquet is helpful for its effective use.

Hemostatic Dressings

When direct pressure is unable to control bleeding, and the injury is located where a tourniquet cannot be applied, you can consider the use of a hemostatic dressing.

A hemostatic dressing is a unique dressing impregnated with an agent that speeds up the clotting process. A hemostatic dressing is packed into an open wound and held in place with direct pressure or a pressure bandage. Pressure is maintained until bleeding has stopped.

Training is essential to learn the proper application of a hemostatic dressing.

Knowledge Check

What is the standard method for controlling external bleeding?

Control of Bleeding

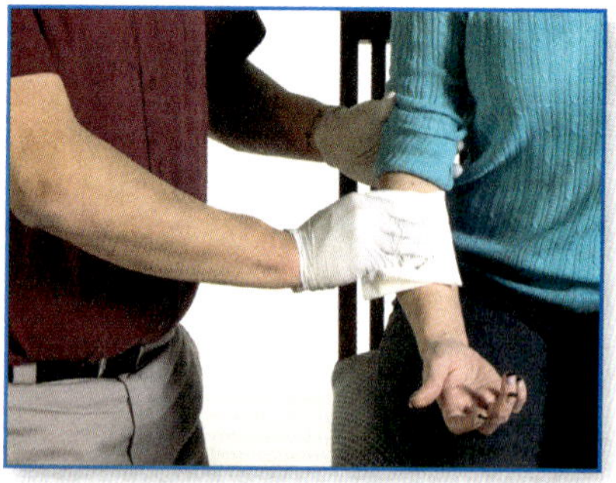

Apply Direct Pressure

- Quickly expose and inspect wound.
- Using a clean pad, apply pressure directly on point of bleeding. Use just gloved hand if pad not available.
- If blood soaks through pad, leave in place. Apply second pad on top of first.
- When controlled, maintain continuous direct pressure.

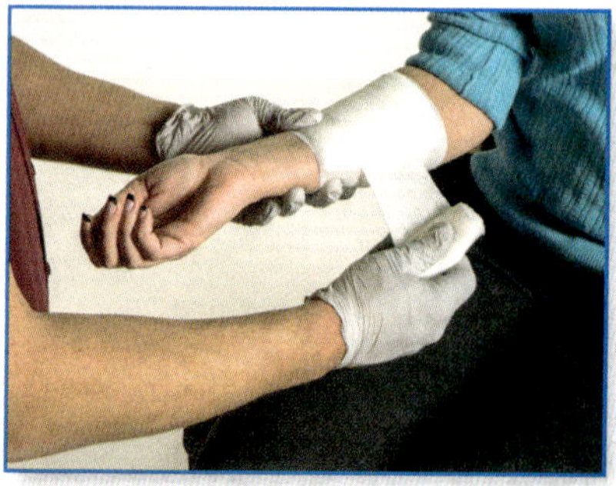

If Bleeding is Controlled

- Consider a pressure bandage. Wrap a conforming bandage around limb and over dressings to provide continuous direct pressure.
- Avoid wrapping so tight that skin beyond bandage becomes cool to the touch or blue in color.

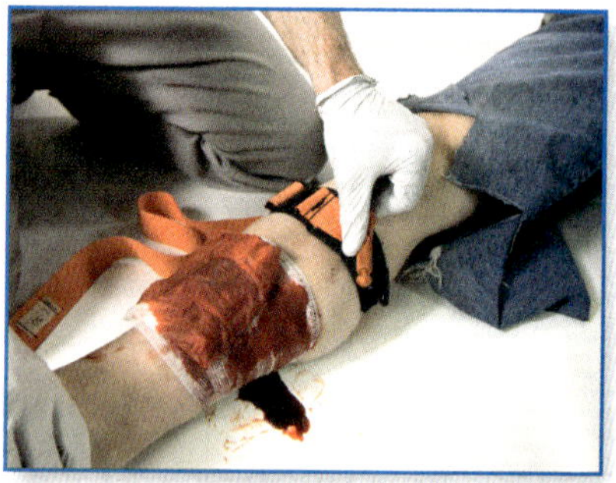

If Bleeding Continues on a Limb

- Apply a commercial tourniquet. If not available, use an improvised one instead.
- Snugly place compressing band a few inches above injury. Twist handle and tighten band until bleeding stops. Secure handle in place.

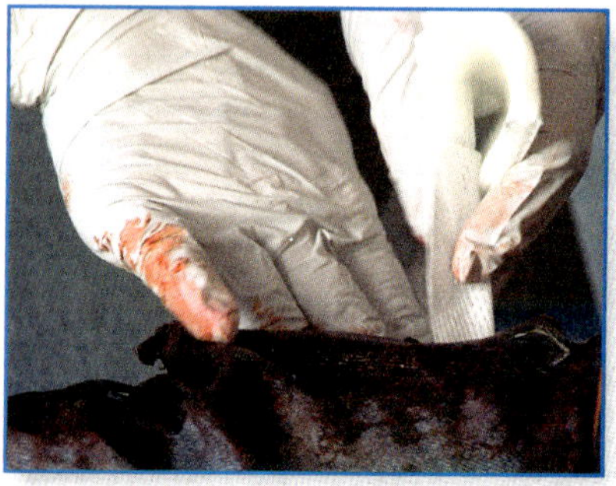

If Bleeding Continues on Torso…

- Consider using a hemostatic dressing if one is available and you are trained to use it.
- Pack dressing tightly into open wound. Place remaining dressing on top of packed wound.
- Secure in place with direct pressure or pressure bandage.

Using a Tourniquet

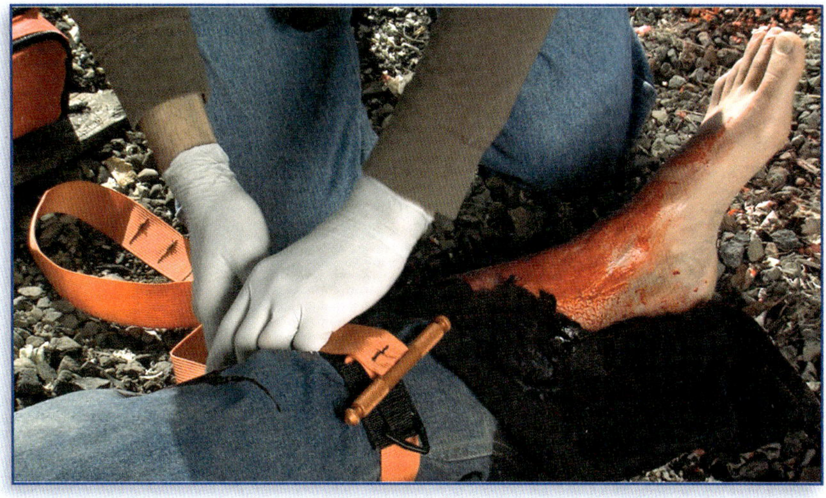

When using a commercial tourniquet, always follow the manufacturer's directions.

Loop the compressing band around the injured limb. If unable to loop it over the limb, unfasten the band, wrap it around the limb, and refasten it. Place the band a few inches above the wound site. Make sure it is not directly over a joint. Hand tighten the band firmly around the limb. Twist the handle to compress the band until bleeding stops. Lock the handle, using the mechanism provided.

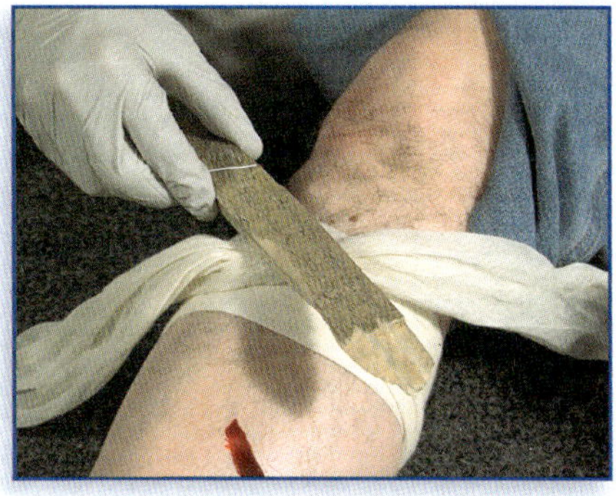

Document the time of application and provide it to EMS personnel. Unless directed by qualified medical personnel, never remove or loosen a tourniquet once it is applied.

To improvise a tourniquet using a triangular bandage, start by folding the bandage lengthwise so that it is approximately 2 inches wide. Place the center of the bandage a few inches above the wound site and not directly over a joint.

Wrap the bandage firmly around the limb, bringing both ends back to the top. Make sure the bandage remains flat. Tie half a knot over the top of the bandage. Place a rigid stick-like object on top of the half-knot and tie a full knot over it. Twist the stick to compress the band until bleeding stops. Secure the stick so it does not loosen or unwind.

Document the time of application and provide it to EMS personnel. As with a commercial tourniquet, do not loosen or remove an improvised tourniquet unless directed by qualified medical personnel.

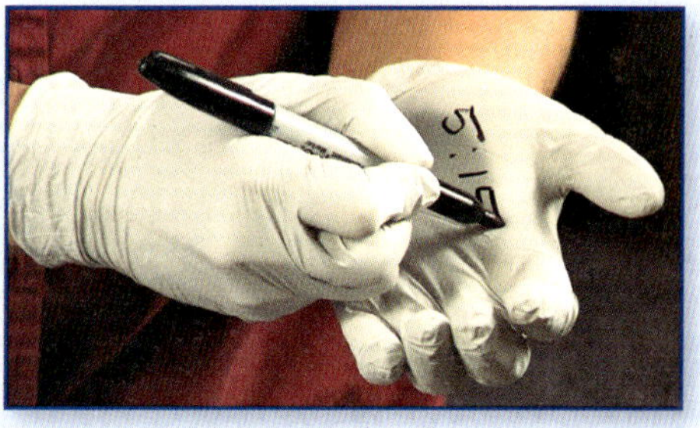

Using a Commercial Tourniquet

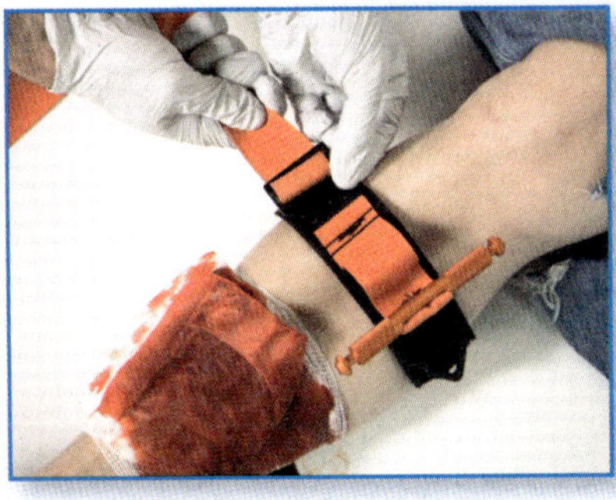

Place Tourniquet

- Loop band around limb. If necessary, unfasten band, wrap it around limb, and refasten it.
- Place band a few inches above wound site and not over a joint.
- Hand-tighten band snugly around limb.

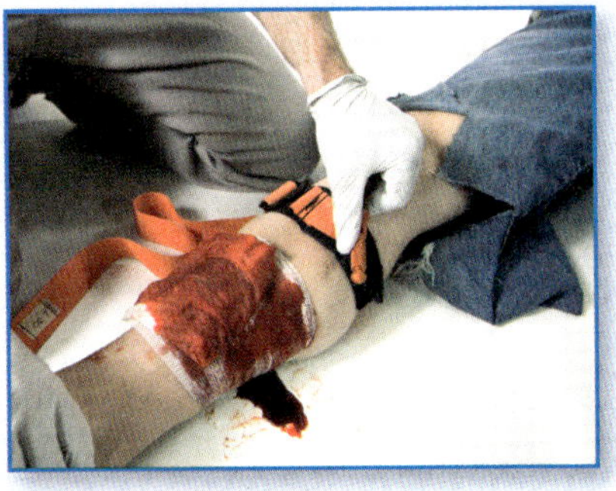

Twist Handle

- Twist handle to compress band around limb.
- Twist until bleeding stops.

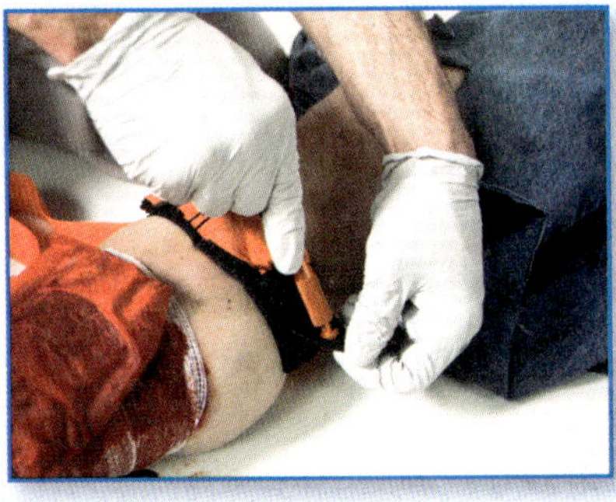

Secure the Handle

- Lock handle in place using mechanism provided to prevent it from loosening or unwinding.

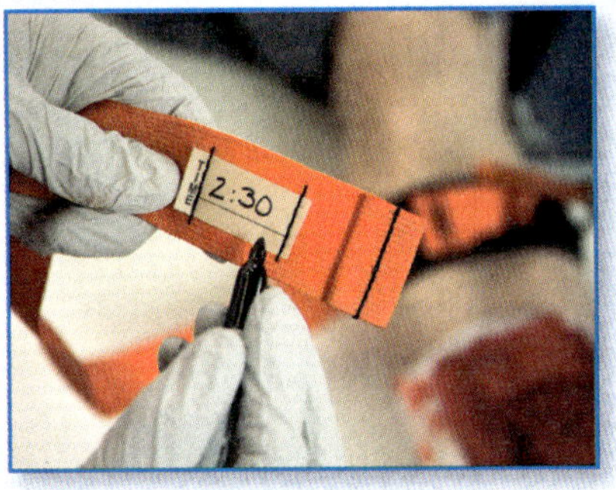

Document Time

- Document time of application and inform EMS personnel when they arrive.
- Do not remove or loosen tourniquet unless directed to by quaified medical personnel.

Using an Improvised Tourniquet

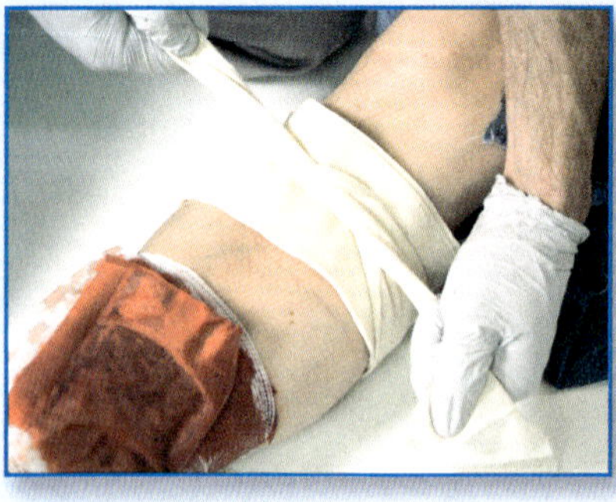

Place Tourniquet

- Fold bandage lengthwise until about 2 inches wide.
- Place center of bandage a few inches above wound site and not over a joint.
- Wrap snugly around limb, bringing both ends back to top. Tie half-knot to keep in place.

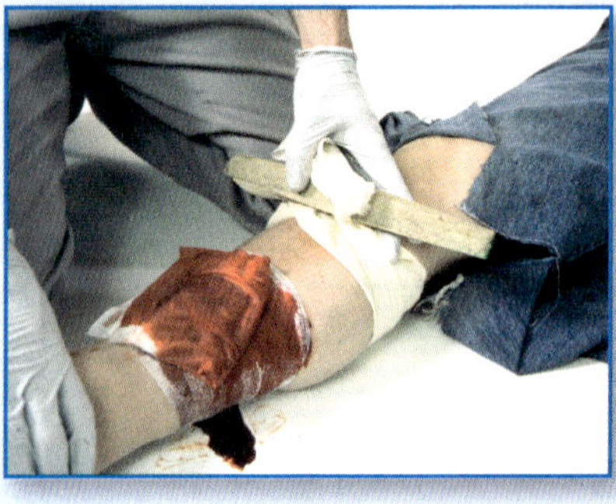

Twist Stick

- Place a rigid stick-like object on top of half knot. Tie full knot over stick.
- Twist stick to compress bandage around limb until bleeding stops.

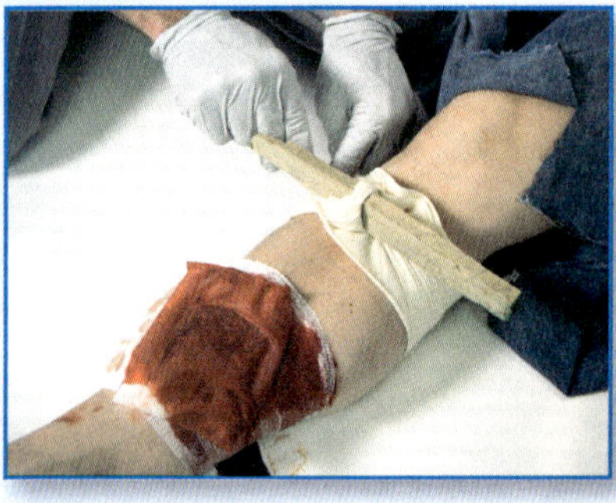

Secure Stick

- Wrap bandage tails around stick to prevent it from loosening or unwinding.

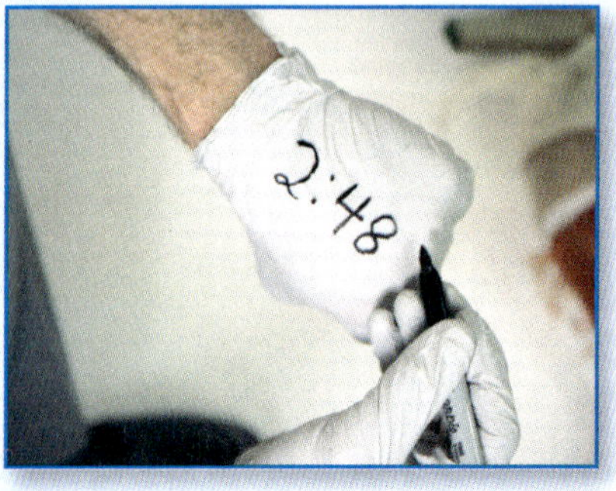

Document Time

- Document time of application and inform EMS personnel when they arrive.
- Do not remove or loosen tourniquet unless directed to by qualified medical personnel.

Using a Hemostatic Dressing

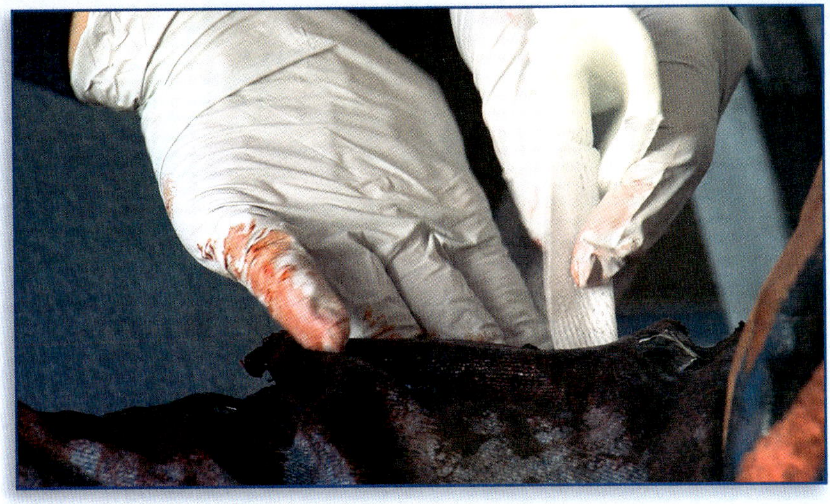

If injury is located where a tourniquet cannot be applied and direct pressure is unable to control bleeding, consider use of a hemostatic dressing.

When using a hemostatic dressing, always follow the manufacturer's directions:

- Remove the dressing from the packaging. The dressing is folded in a Z pattern to help with proper use.
- Pull end of dressing out from one side and pack into wound, directly over the source of bleeding.
- When the wound is packed, apply direct pressure using the rest of the dressing. Continue to apply pressure until bleeding stops.
- Consider using direct pressure or a pressure bandage over the wound to maintain bleeding control.

Using Hemostatic Dressings

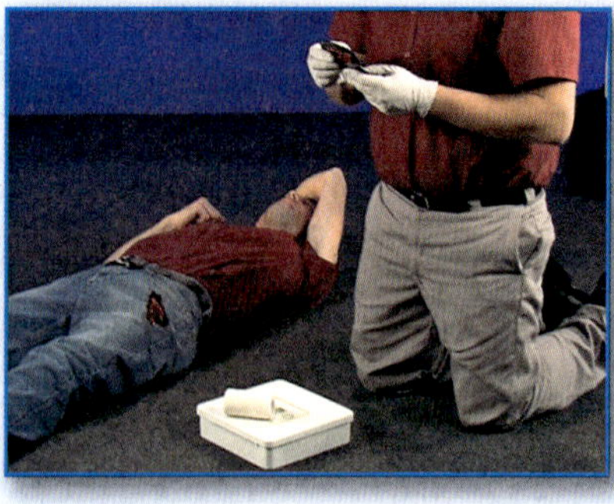

Assess Injury

- If injury is located where a tourniquet cannot be applied and direct pressure is unable to control bleeding, consider use of a hemostatic dressing.

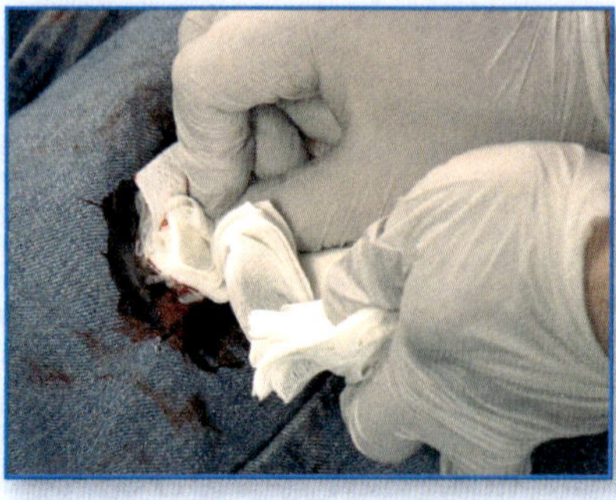

Pack Dressing into Wound

- Remove the dressing from packaging; dressing is folded in a Z pattern to help with proper use.
- Pull end of dressing out from one side and pack into wound, directly over source of bleeding.

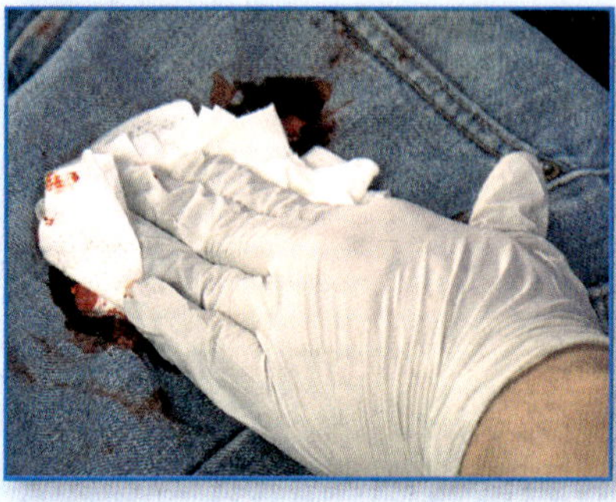

Apply Direct Pressure

- When wound is tightly packed apply direct pressure over wound site using remaining part of dressing. Continue to apply pressure until bleeding stops.
- If bleeding is controlled, consider using a pressure bandage to hold dressing in place.

Shock

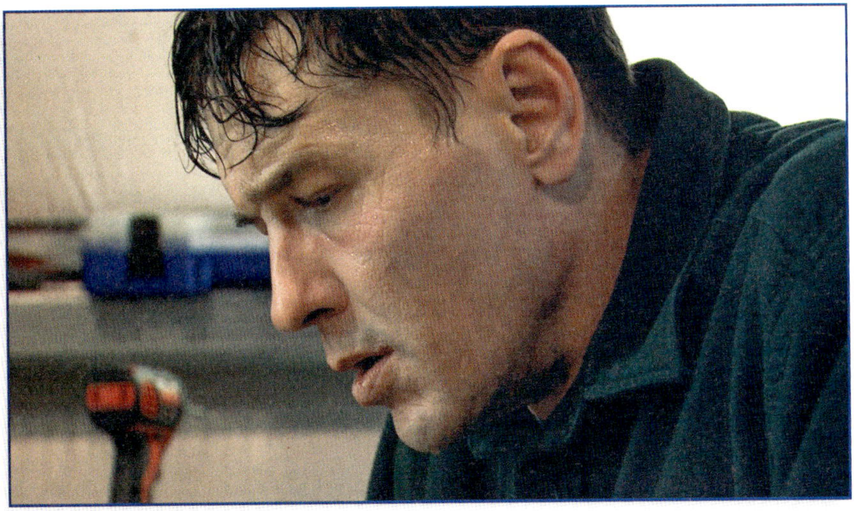

Shock develops when poor blood flow creates a shortage of oxygen to body tissues. Any serious illness or injury has the potential to cause shock. If not treated early, it can get worse and become life threatening.

Early signs can be difficult to detect. A person may simply begin to appear uneasy, restless, or worried. Other, more serious signs can emerge gradually. The person may become confused. The skin may become pale, cool, and sweaty.

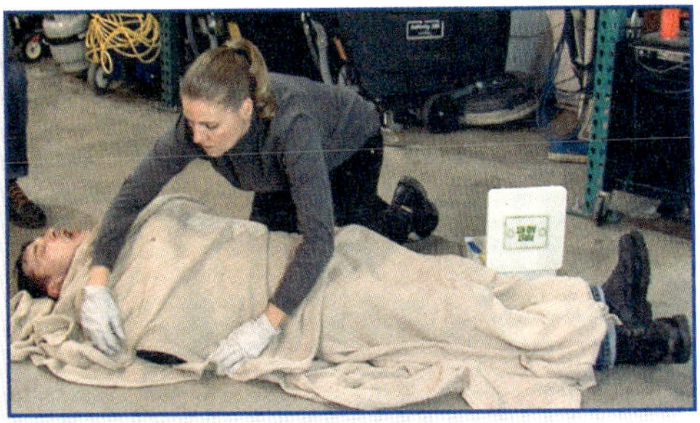

A person in shock must get to a hospital as quickly as possible. Early recognition, treatment, and activation of EMS are essential for survival.

To limit the effects of shock, help the body maintain adequate oxygen by ensuring an open and clear airway, confirming normal breathing, and controlling any external bleeding. If there is no difficulty in breathing, lay the person flat on the ground.

Maintain a normal body temperature. Insulate on top and underneath to prevent heat loss. Be careful not to overheat. Give nothing to eat or drink, even if the person asks for it. Keep the person as comfortable and calm as possible. Reassess regularly until another provider or EMS take over.

Internal Bleeding

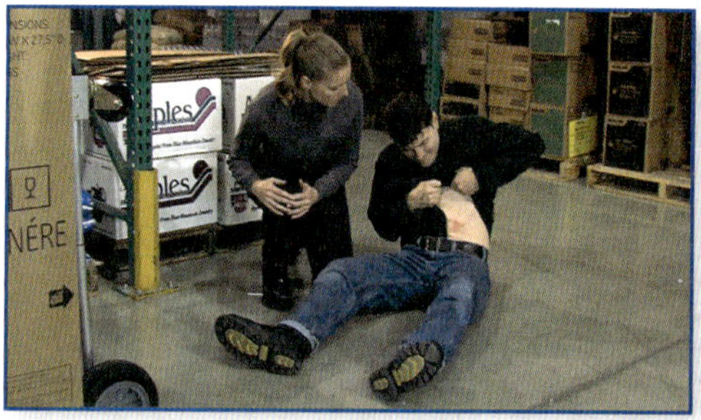

A significant blow can create injury and bleeding inside the body. This is especially true for blood vessels and organs in the chest and abdomen. Because you cannot clearly see the injury, internal bleeding can be difficult to detect. Suspect it if the chest or abdomen was hit hard. Signs of shock may be the earliest indication that internal bleeding is occurring.

Knowledge Check

At the elementary school where you teach, one of your students tells you that another child fell off the play structure at recess. Concerned, you approach the child who fell and ask her what happened. She tells you she hit her belly on one of the bars when she fell and that it hurt a lot at first, but that it feels better now. You are concerned whether she injured herself internally. What signs do you look for?

Amputation

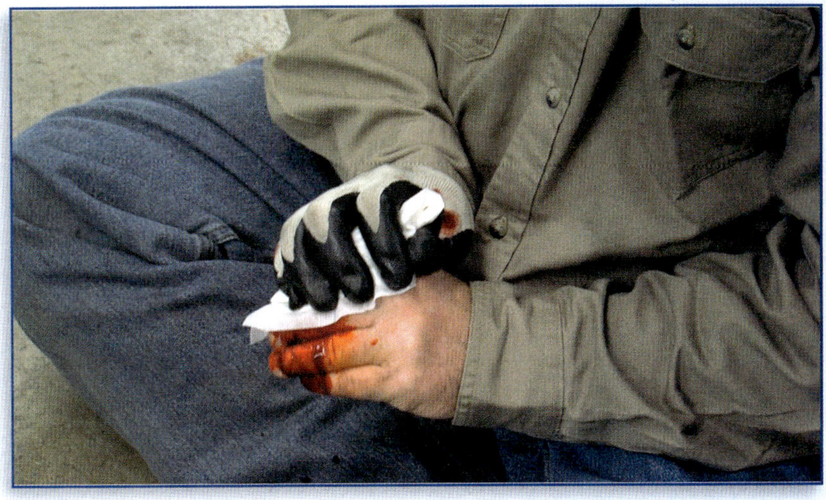

Amputation is the complete detachment of a body part. If an amputation has occurred, quickly assess for and control any severe bleeding. Have the person sit or lie down, even if it is on the ground. Activate EMS.

Amputated body parts can often be surgically reattached. Once the person is stable, locate the severed part. Wrap it in a sterile or clean cloth. Place the part in a tightly sealed plastic bag or waterproof container. If available, cool the bag or container with ice or a chemical cold pack.

Do not soak the severed part in water, and do not put it directly on ice. Give it to EMS providers for transport with the person to the hospital.

Calm, comfort, and reassure the person. Reassess regularly until another provider or EMS take over.

Knowledge Check

True or false? Quickly assessing for and controlling any bleeding is the highest priority if an amputation has occurred.

Impaled Objects

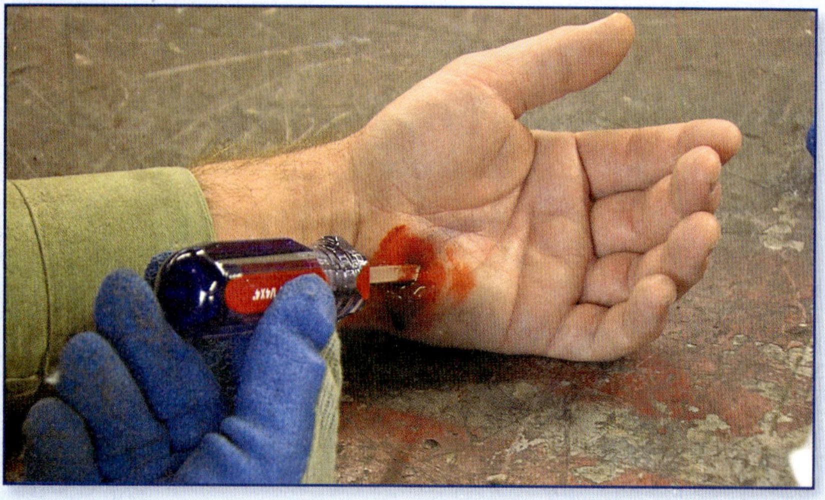

An impaled object is an object that penetrates a body part and remains embedded. As a general rule, do not remove an impaled object. If it has damaged any large blood vessels, it can act like a plug, helping to prevent serious blood loss.

Movement of the object, or the body part it is in, could also create additional injury, especially if the object is embedded in muscle, bone, or organs below the skin.

If you suspect impalement has occurred, carefully tear or cut away clothing to confirm the object has penetrated the skin. Look for any serious bleeding.

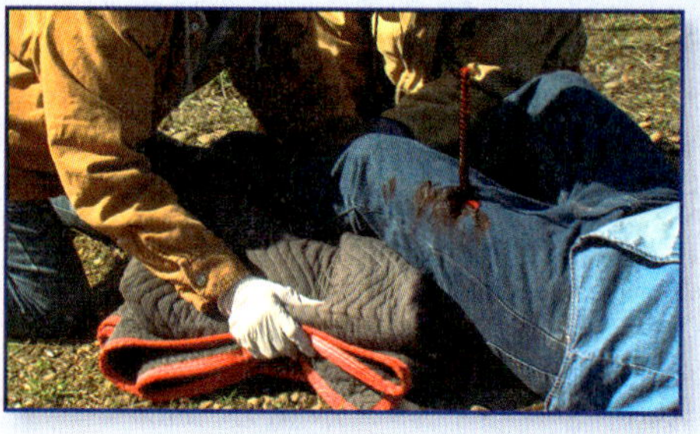

Keep the affected body part immobilized to prevent movement. Activate EMS for any significant impaled object or if you are in doubt about its severity. If the injury is bleeding, use clean pads to apply direct pressure straight down around the base of the object to control it. Do not apply pressure to the object itself.

To prevent movement of the object, place bulkier padding around it for stabilization. Hold the padding in place with your gloved hand or a bandage.

Being impaled on a larger, more immovable object requires additional care. If needed, support the person's weight to relieve pressure on the impalement. Use padding to provide stability and comfort. Reassure the person to keep him or her calm. Make him or her as comfortable as possible. Reassess the person and the injury regularly until EMS personnel can take over care.

Impaled Object in the Eye

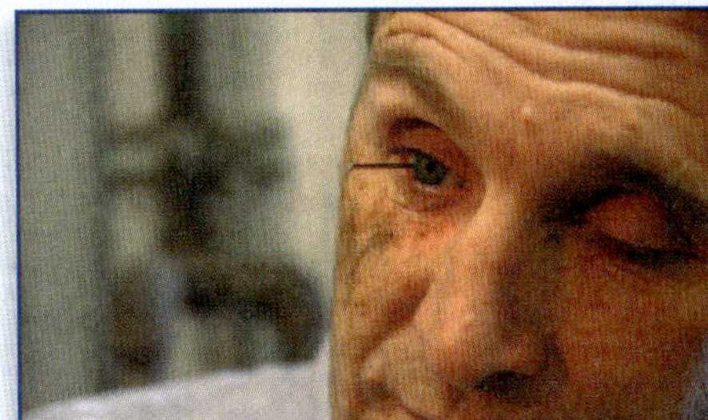

The impalement of an unprotected eye is most likely to be caused by a small object being propelled at a high rate of speed.

Activate EMS. Prompt professional medical care is required anytime an object penetrates the surface of the eye. The immediate focus of care is to stabilize the object and prevent additional injury. Do not allow the person to rub the eye. Never try to remove an embedded object.

Stabilize a large object with clean pads. Place a protective cover over the object, such as a paper cup or cone. Cover the uninjured eye with a pad and bandage over both eyes. With smaller objects, loosely cover both eyes with pads and bandage. Eyes move together. Covering both eyes prevents movement of the affected eye.

Covering both eyes can be distressing. Stay with the person. Calm, comfort, and reassure to help reduce anxiety. Regularly assess the person until EMS personnel take over.

Knowledge Check

Another carpenter with whom you work has accidently driven a framing nail into his hand with a nail gun. The nail is embedded deeply and extends out the other side of his hand. As a first aid trained provider, you begin to provide care. You elect to leave the impaled nail in place. What are the two main reasons you make that decision?

Open Chest Injury

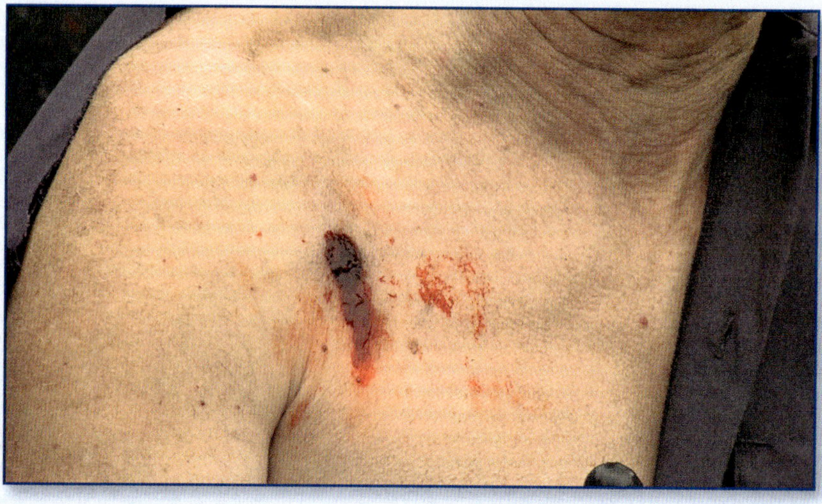

A penetrating injury through the chest wall can disrupt the chest's ability to draw air into the lungs. Expansion of the chest during breathing creates suction in the chest, which pulls outside air containing oxygen through the airway and into the lungs. An open wound on the chest wall will also allow air to be drawn into the chest. This will get progressively worse over time and significantly impair breathing. The person's condition could deteriorate quickly.

Activate EMS immediately. Remove clothing to expose the injury site to assess the wound. Check to see if there is an exit injury on the other side of the chest. If so, treat the more serious one first. Do not seal the open wound with an airtight dressing. If you do, pressure within the chest could increase and quickly become life threatening. Be careful that your bleeding control measures do not unintentionally seal the wound.

If possible, allow the person to assume a position he or she is most comfortable breathing in. Regularly assess the person and the injury until EMS providers assume care. Be prepared to perform CPR if breathing stops.

Knowledge Check

True or false? It is recommended that first aid providers seal an open chest wound with an airtight dressing.

Open Abdominal Injury

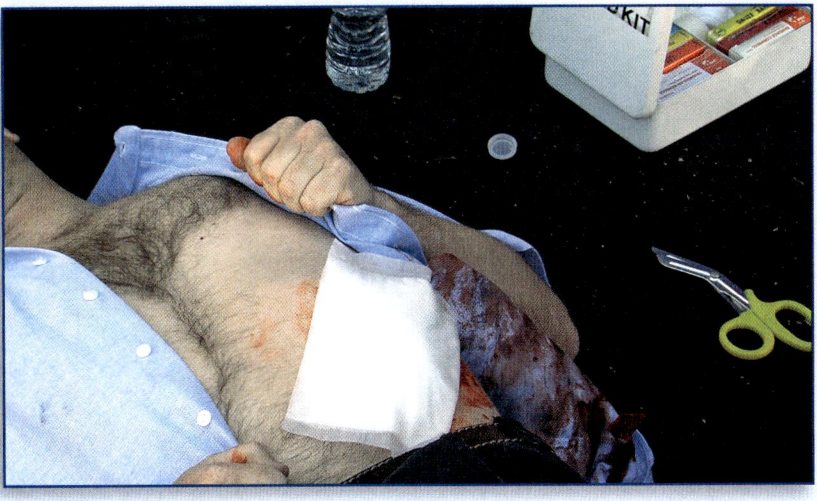

Injury to the abdomen may result in a condition known as evisceration, in which abdominal organs protrude through an open wound. It is important to understand that these are functioning organs and the primary treatment is to protect them from further injury.

Activate EMS. Allow the person to assume a position of comfort. Cover any protruding organs with a thick, moist dressing. Do not push the organs back inside the body. Do not apply direct pressure on the wound or exposed internal parts, as this could cause further injury.

Regularly assess the person and the injury until EMS personnel arrive and take over care.

Knowledge Check

Your fellow cook at a restaurant is doing prep work when she slips while trimming a large piece of meat. She accidentally draws a sharp knife blade across the abdomen, cutting through the abdominal wall. As a trained first aid provider, you cut away her shirt to expose and inspect the wound. It is not bleeding very much but you see abdominal organs protruding through the open wound. Knowing these are functioning organs, how are you going to protect them from further injury?

Head, Neck, or Back Injury

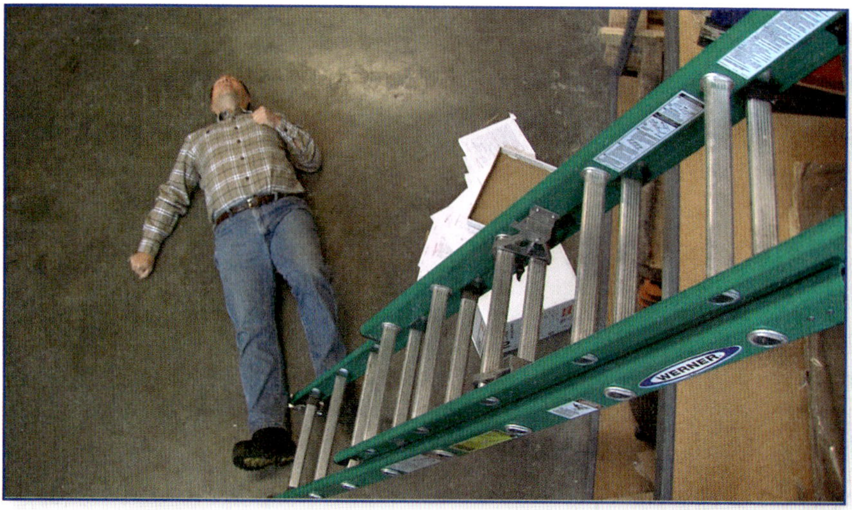

The head, neck, and back are all vulnerable when the body experiences a sudden force.

Spinal Injury

When the body suffers a significant force, such as from a high fall, shooting, or motor vehicle crash, serious injury can result, most notably to the spine. Injury to the spinal cord can result in temporary or permanent paralysis. Paralysis of chest muscles could result in the loss of breathing. Serious shock may also occur.

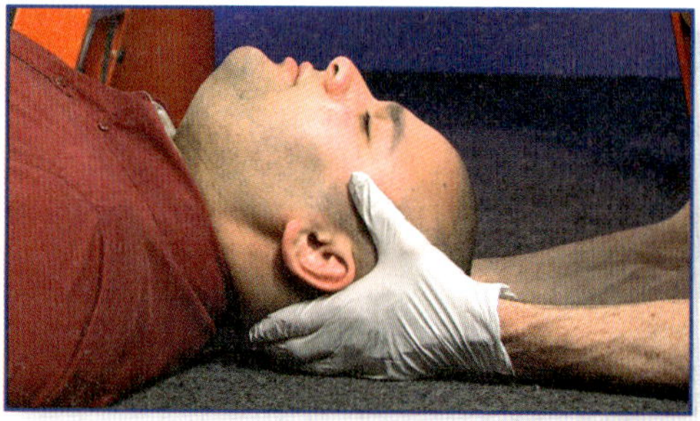

After an initial injury, the movement of damaged spinal bones can result in additional injury to the spinal cord or surrounding tissue.

Suspect a spinal injury when the following occur:

- Obvious injuries to head, neck, or back
- Numbness, tingling, burning, or a loss of sensation in the arms, hands, legs, or feet

The lack of symptoms or obvious injury does not mean that the spine is not injured. If a significant mechanism of injury occurred, it is best to assume a spinal injury exists. Manually stabilize the head in place with your hands to provide spinal motion restriction.

Establishing an airway for an unresponsive person is a higher priority than protecting a suspected injury to the spine. Tilt the head and lift the chin when necessary to maintain an open airway or give rescue breaths.

When a head, neck, or back injury is suspected, it is best to leave the person in the position found. However, if the airway is threatened, quickly roll the person as needed to clear and protect it. Keep the head, shoulders, and torso from twisting as best you can.

If you need to leave an unresponsive person with a suspected spinal injury alone to get help, place the person in a recovery position to protect the airway before you go.

Brain Injury

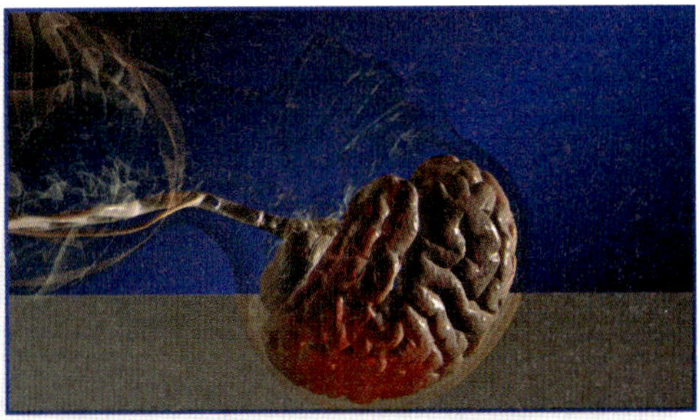

Injury to the brain can occur from a significant blow to the head or by rapid movements of the head that force the brain to bounce around within the skull. Significant swelling or bleeding inside the skull can result in increased pressure that damages delicate brain tissue.

Suspect serious brain injury when a blow to the head clearly results in a diminished level of responsiveness. Surgical intervention may be the only treatment. Activate EMS without delay and stabilize the head with your hands. Do not attempt to stop the flow of blood or fluid from the ears or nose.

If the person has a seizure, protect the head as much as possible and prevent him or her from bumping into nearby objects. Do not restrain the person tightly and do not place anything in his or her mouth. Seizures will generally last for just a few minutes. When the seizure stops, assess the person's breathing and ability to respond. Provide CPR if necessary. Reassess regularly until EMS personnel take over.

Concussion

A concussion is a brain injury that generally results in less immediate or obvious signs. Most concussions are temporary and resolve naturally, but it is possible for one to progress into a life-threatening condition.

Suspect a concussion after a significant blow to the head or body when the affected person is unable to remember what happened just before or after the incident, or recall simple facts about it. The person may move clumsily, answer questions slowly, or show a change in mood or personality. Additional signs include the following:

- Looking stunned or dazed
- Headache
- Nausea
- Dizziness
- Difficulty in balance
- Visual problems

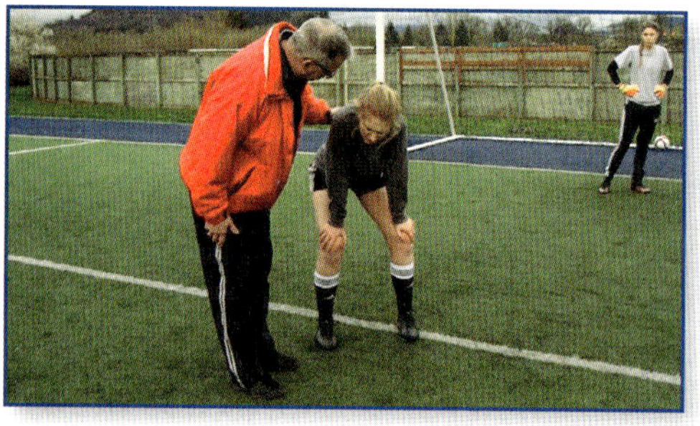

A first aid provider may be called upon to give advice on whether someone who may have a concussion is okay to return to normal activities. Unfortunately, there is no current concussion evaluation process for use by those trained in first aid.

If you suspect a concussion may have occurred, the affected person should be evaluated by a healthcare provider or EMS personnel as soon as possible.

Because of the potential progressive nature of concussion, it is best to not allow the person to perform actions that could pose a risk for additional injury until he or she can be adequately assessed by a healthcare professional.

Knowledge Check

You are driving along your delivery route when you witness one car hitting another car at a high rate of speed. Trained as a first aid provider, you stop to help. The scene is secured and the driver of the car you have gone to help has no immediate life threats that you can assess. However, she is not wearing a seat belt and it appears she was thrown forward into the windshield, hitting it with her head. There is a small cut on her forehead, but she does not complain of pain in her neck, or numbness and tingling in her arms or legs. You elect to manually stabilize her head with your hands. Why?

Manual Spinal Motion Restriction

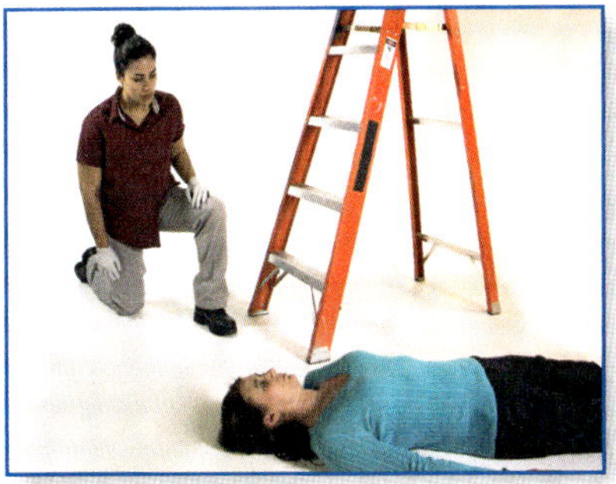

Initial Considerations

- Make sure it is safe to provide care.
- Immediately encourage person to not move.
- Have a bystander activate EMS.

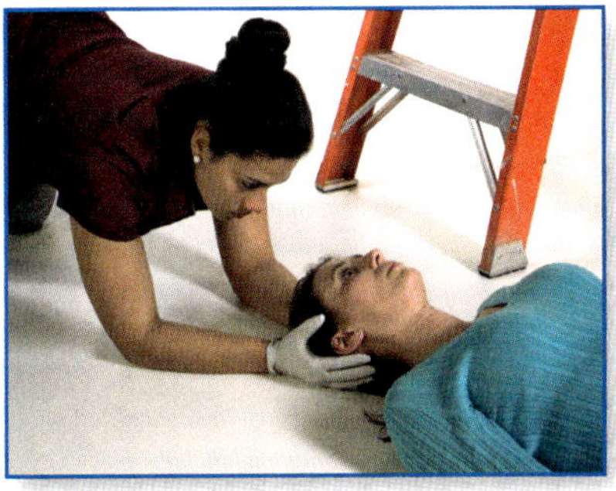

Stabilize Head

- Get into a comfortable position behind person.
- Cup your hands on both sides of head, to manually stabilize it.
- Minimize any motion.
- Comfort, calm, and reassure person.

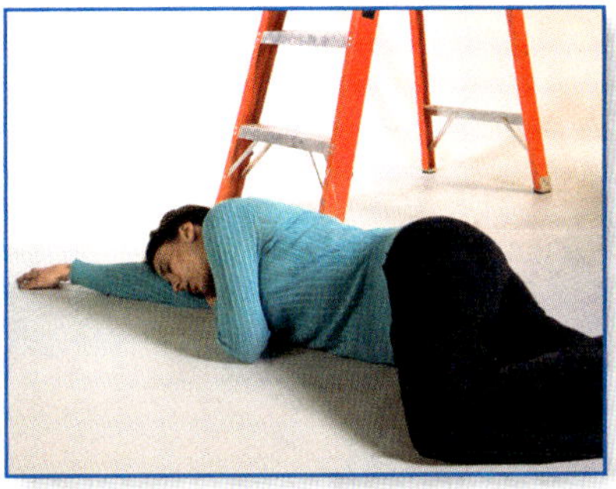

Protect Airway

- If fluids are collecting in mouth and airway, roll person onto side to drain.
- If you are alone and need to leave to get help, roll person into recovery position before you go.

Swollen, Painful, or Deformed Limb

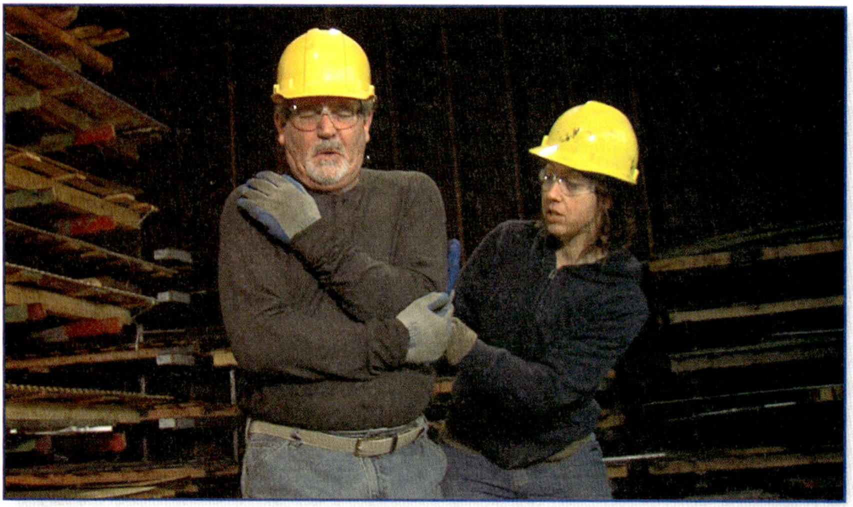

Bones, muscles, and joints give the body shape, allow movement, and protect vital internal organs. Long bones form the upper and lower parts of each limb. Muscles, ligaments, and tendons attach to the bones, allowing for movement where the bones come together at joints. These bones are the most exposed to external forces and injury.

There are four different types of injuries affecting bones, muscles, and joints:

- Strains are stretching or tearing injuries to muscles or tendons.
- Sprains are tearing injuries to ligaments that hold joints together.
- Dislocations are the separation of bone ends at a joint.
- Fractures are breaks in bones.

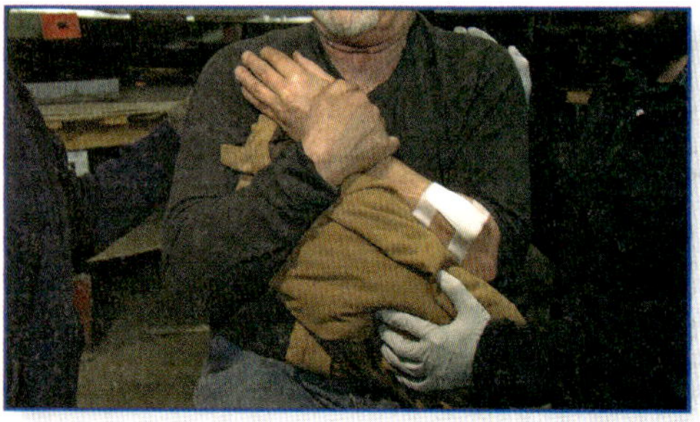

Common signs of these types of injuries include swelling, pain, and discoloration. Distinguishing the exact type of injury is often difficult. It is best to treat everything as a possible fracture.

The limb may appear deformed and the person may guard it by holding it against his or her body. Unstable bones or joints can damage surrounding tissue. Encourage the person to not move or use the injured limb. If the injury seems serious, or you are not sure, activate EMS.

It is best to not straighten an injured limb that is unnaturally angled. Leave the limb in the position found. If a limb becomes blue or extremely pale, circulation may be compromised by the injury. Activate EMS if this occurs.

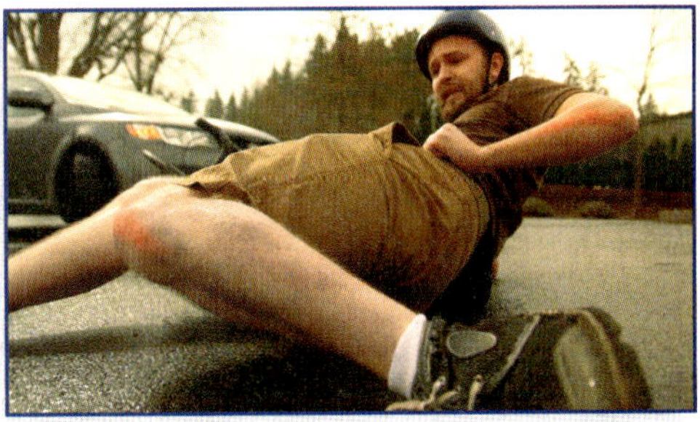

Splinting an injured limb can reduce pain and prevent further injury, especially when moving an injured person. In general, it is best to rely on EMS personnel to splint, as they have more extensive training, experience, and equipment.

Comfort, calm, and reassure the person. Reassess the person and injury regularly until EMS personnel take over.

Local Cooling

For many injuries, local cooling can help decrease bleeding, swelling, and pain. A plastic bag filled with a mixture of ice and water works best. Place a thin cloth between the bag and skin to prevent cold-related problems. Limit application to 20 minutes or less.

Knowledge Check

One of your coworkers was hit in the leg with a wide load on a forklift. As a responding first aid provider, you carefully cut her pant leg open to expose the injury site and find the lower leg is lying at an unnatural angle and the tissue color of the leg and foot below the injury is a grayish blue. What do you do?

Manual Stabilization of a Limb

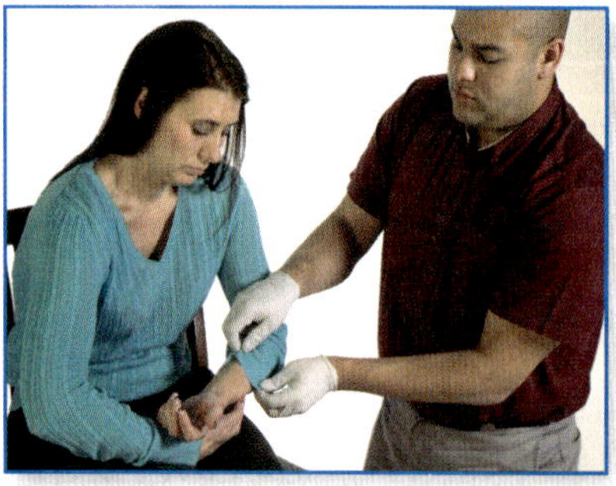

Expose Injury

- Encourage person not to move injured limb.
- Expose injury site to look for an open wound.

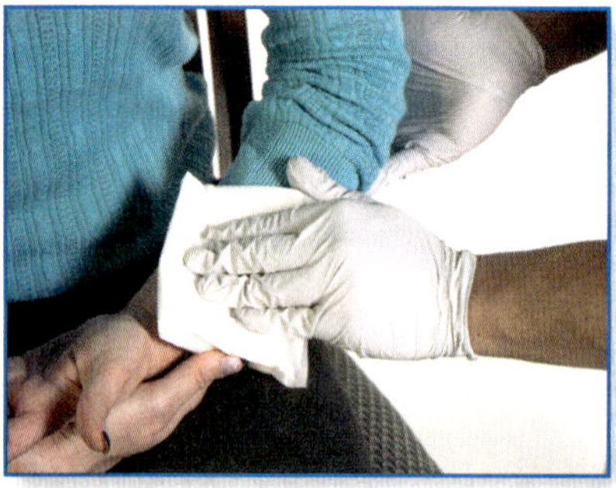

Cover Open Wounds

- Cover an open wound with a clean absorbent pad.
- Gently control bleeding with firm, continuous, direct pressure around bone or injury site.
- Never push an exposed bone back under skin.

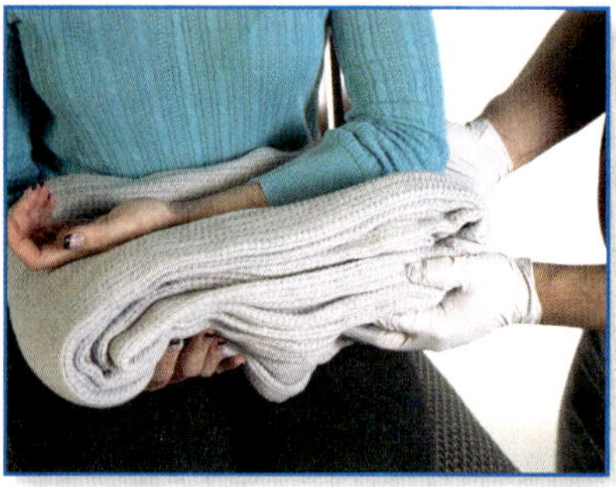

Stabilize Limb

- Leave injured limb in position it was found.
- Use padding in gaps and holes underneath limb to provide a stable and comfortable spot for it to rest.
- If needed, use your hands to manually stabilize limb.

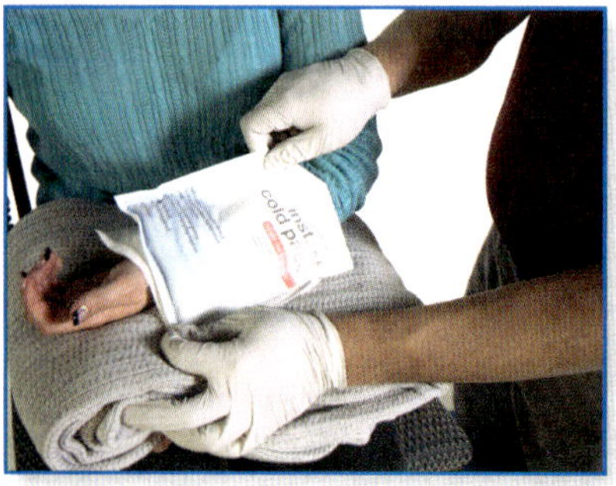

Additional Considerations

- If injury seems serious, or you are not sure, activate EMS.
- Comfort, calm, and reassure person.
- Local cooling can help decrease bleeding, swelling, and pain.

Burns

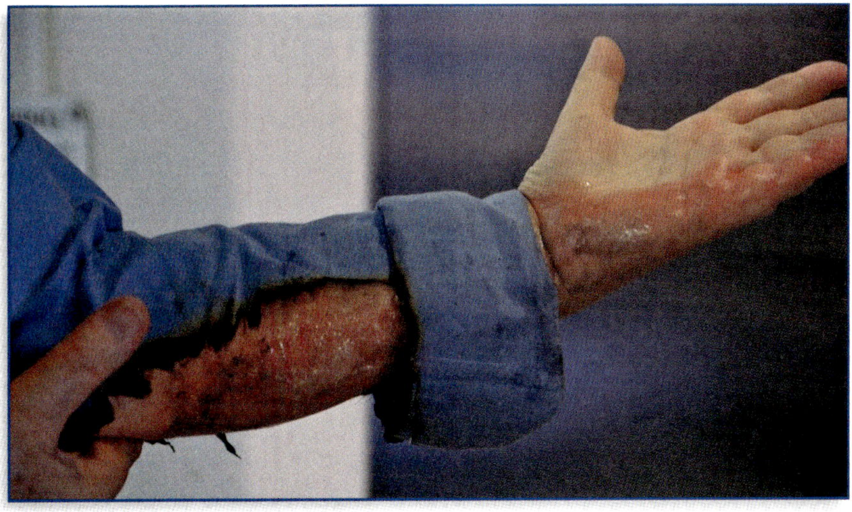

A burn is an injury to skin, and possibly underlying tissues, caused by exposure to extreme heat, chemicals, or electrical contact.

Thermal Burns

Common causes of thermal burns include direct contact with hot liquids, flames, or hot objects. Burns can also be caused by radiant heat from a hot environment or extended exposure to the sun. Most burns are minor in nature and may only require basic care. However, more serious burns require additional care.

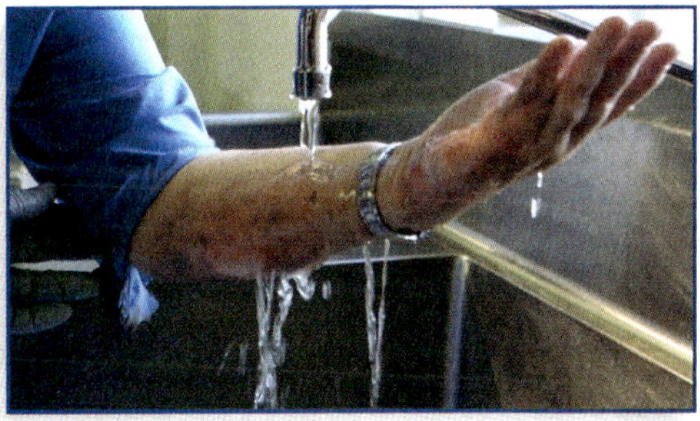

The severity of a burn is related to its depth and size. Deeper burns resulting in blistering or broken skin are more serious. Larger burns, even those with a shallow depth, are also more serious. Burn location contributes to severity. Burns involving the face, neck, hands, genitals, and feet can result in complications related to movement and other basic functions. Difficulty breathing as a result of inhaling hot air indicates a serious injury within the airway. All serious burns, or ones you are unsure about, should be evaluated by a healthcare provider.

When a burn occurs, make sure the situation is safe for you to help. If clothes or other materials are burning or on fire, act immediately to put the fire out.

Direct a person to stop, drop, and roll. Smother the burning material with a coat, rug, or blanket, or douse the material with water.

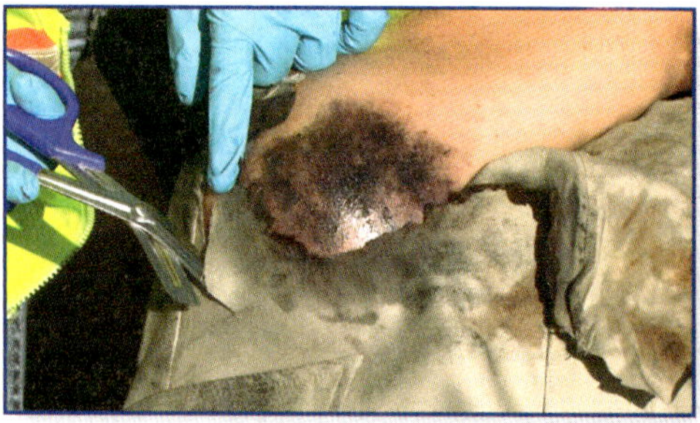

Activate EMS if you think the burn is severe or you are unsure. Carefully expose burned areas by removing clothing. If needed, cut or tear clothing away. If it is stuck to the burn, cut around it. Cool a burn with cool or cold water as quickly as possible. Cool the burn for at least 10 minutes. Use a clean, cool or cold dressing as an alternative when water is not available. Never use ice or a frozen compress to cool a burn. There are also gel-soaked burn dressings, presoaked with a specially formulated gel, to promote cooling of the burn.

Early cooling can reduce pain and minimize the risk and depth of burn injury. When cooling large burns, watch for signs of overcooling, such as shivering. Children have a larger surface area in relation to weight than adults and are more likely to have complications from overcooling.

Remove any jewelry near the burned area. After cooling, separate fingers or toes with sterile dressings or pads. To improve healing, leave any blisters intact. Loosely cover the burn area with a dry, clean pad or clean sheet to help keep it clean and protected. Avoid natural burn remedies such as honey or potato peels. Never apply butter, ointment, lotion, or antiseptic to a serious burn. Give the person nothing to eat or drink. Keep the person calm and comfortable while awaiting EMS.

Electrical Burns

Medical emergencies involving electricity can occur when there is direct contact with an energized object, such as an electrical wire or outlet, or when someone is struck by lightning.

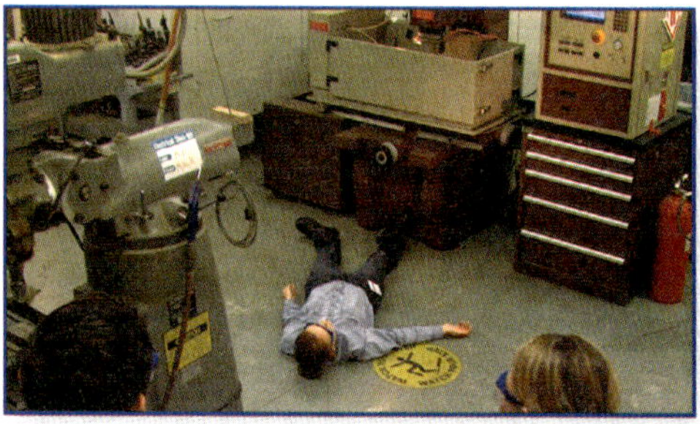

Be safe! Turn off any electrical current before touching the person. If you cannot stop the flow of electricity, do not enter the area around the person or attempt to care for him or her.

An electric shock can cause an abnormal heart rhythm in which the heart stops moving blood. When it is safe, perform CPR and use an AED if one becomes available.

When a body part comes into contact with an exposed electrical source, electricity can travel from the point of contact to a second point of contact that is grounded. Common points of contact include the hands and the feet.

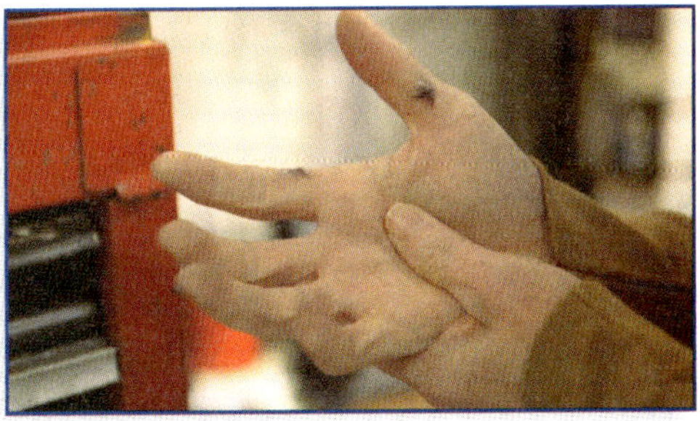

If the person affected is responsive and no longer in contact with the electrical source, look for burns at any suspected points of contact. Cool the burn as you would with a thermal burn.

A person who has received an electrical shock should seek professional medical care because serious internal injuries can occur.

CAUTION!

Consider any fallen or broken wire extremely dangerous. Do not touch (or allow your clothing to touch) a wire, person, or vehicle that is possibly energized. Do not approach within 8 feet of it. Notify the local utility and have trained personnel sent to scene. NEVER attempt to handle wires yourself unless you are properly trained and equipped.

Chemical Burns

Some chemicals can damage skin tissue on contact. The priority is to quickly remove the chemical to minimize any damage. Immediately flood the affected area with large amounts of water. Take care to prevent additional exposure to the injured person or yourself.

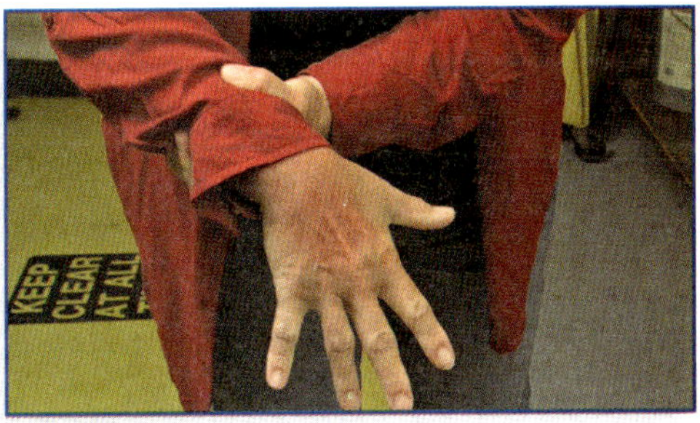

When involved, brush off any dry powder with a gloved hand or cloth prior to flushing. Do this carefully to avoid additional exposure.

Carefully remove any contaminated clothing while continuing to flush the area. Flush for at least 15 minutes. Some chemicals take longer than others to be flushed away. If still painful, resume flushing. If no longer painful, cover any visible burns loosely with a dry, clean dressing and seek further medical attention.

Chemicals in the Eye

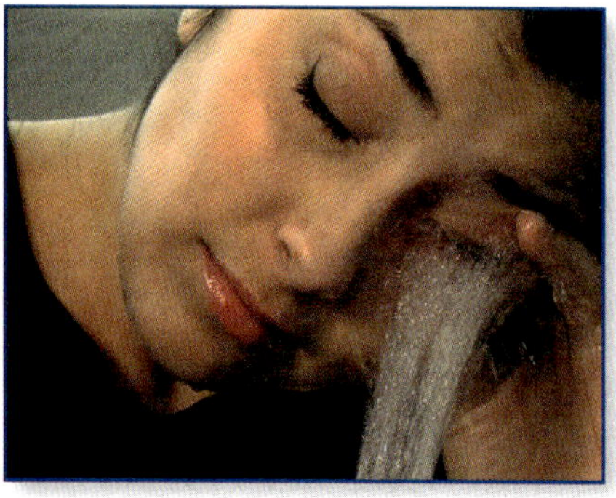

Corrosive chemicals splashed into an eye can quickly damage eye tissue. Affected eyes will become painful and appear red and watery. Immediately flood the eye with large amounts of water. Carefully hold the eye open and flush continuously for at least 15 minutes, or until EMS personnel take over.

Flush outward from the nose side of the affected eye to prevent contamination of an unaffected eye. If the person is wearing contact lenses and they are not removed by the flushing, have the person try to remove them as flushing continues. If running water is not available, normal saline or another commercial eye irrigating solution can be used.

Chemical burns to the eye require professional medical care. Activate EMS as quickly as possible.

Without interrupting care, contact the Poison Help line at 1-800-222-1222 for treatment advice when a chemical burn occurs. If not available, talk to the EMS dispatcher or a medical provider.

Knowledge Check

A nearby coworker using a torch to free up a stuck bolt accidentally ignites his shirt sleeve on fire. As a trained first aid provider, you quickly put out the flames by throwing a nearby coat over his arm. When you remove the coat, you can see that his arm has been burned badly. What is your next step to remove heat from the burned area and prevent additional damage?

Minor Injuries

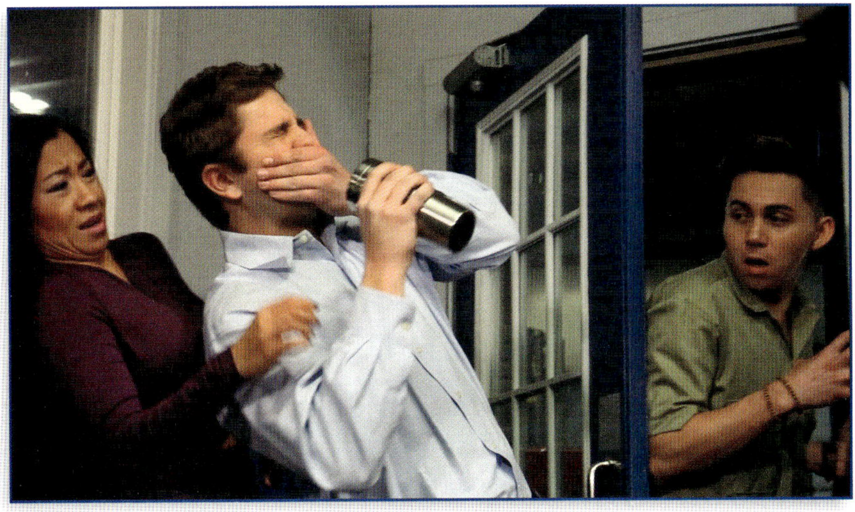

Minor injuries, which can also be sudden and surprising, may need first aid attention.

Nosebleed

Nosebleeds can occur when small blood vessels inside the nostrils are ruptured. Most nosebleeds are not serious and can be easily handled.

To care for someone with a nosebleed, have the person sit up straight with his or her head tilted forward, chin down. Pinch the soft portion of the nose with your thumb and index finger and hold it for about ten minutes. Do not tilt the head back or have the person lie down. These actions will cause the person to swallow blood and may cause him or her to vomit. Have the person spit out any blood that collects in his or her mouth.

Monitor the person. If the nose continues to bleed, or you see signs of developing shock, seek further medical help.

Injured Tooth

A blow to the mouth can break, dislocate, or even knock out teeth. When a tooth has been knocked out, treat it without delay. Immediate reimplantation is believed by the dental community to result in the greatest chance of tooth survival.

Control any bleeding. Have the person gently bite down on a clean absorbent pad over the bleeding socket. Handle the tooth only by the chewing surface, called the crown. Do not touch the root, the part of the tooth that extends into the gum. Never scrub the tooth or remove any attached tissue fragments.

Keeping the tooth moist can help extend the time for successful reimplantation. At a minimum, have the person spit into a cup and place the tooth in the saliva. Avoid storage in water.

There are alternative solutions that are more effective for temporary storage of a displaced tooth than saliva:

- Hank's Balanced Salt Solution
- Propolis
- Egg white
- Coconut water
- Ricetral
- Whole milk

Get the person to a dentist as quickly as possible, within an hour. The faster you act, the better the chance of saving the tooth.

Splinter

Splinters are small, sharp pieces of foreign material that become embedded in the skin. They need to be removed to keep a wound from becoming inflamed or infected.

Most splinters can be easily treated. If there is a protruding end, use tweezers to grab the splinter and pull it out in the direction it entered. Following use, tweezers should be washed thoroughly with soap and water.

If a splinter is deeply embedded or you have only been able to remove a piece of it, seek professional medical care.

Irritated Eyes

Small foreign objects on the surface of an eye will cause irritation and discomfort.

Encourage the person not to rub the affected eye. Have the person blink several times to see if the eyelid or tearing can remove the object naturally. If not, flush the eye with tap water or saline eyewash solution. Flush outward from the nose side of the eye.

If pain continues or the person feels like something is still in the eye, cover the eye lightly with a gauze pad and seek professional medical care. If the person has been exposed to flying metal fragments (hammering, grinding, etc.), do not attempt removal. Seek professional medical care immediately.

Knowledge Check

When a tooth has been knocked out, what is the most critical factor in being able to successfully reimplant the tooth?

Sudden Illness

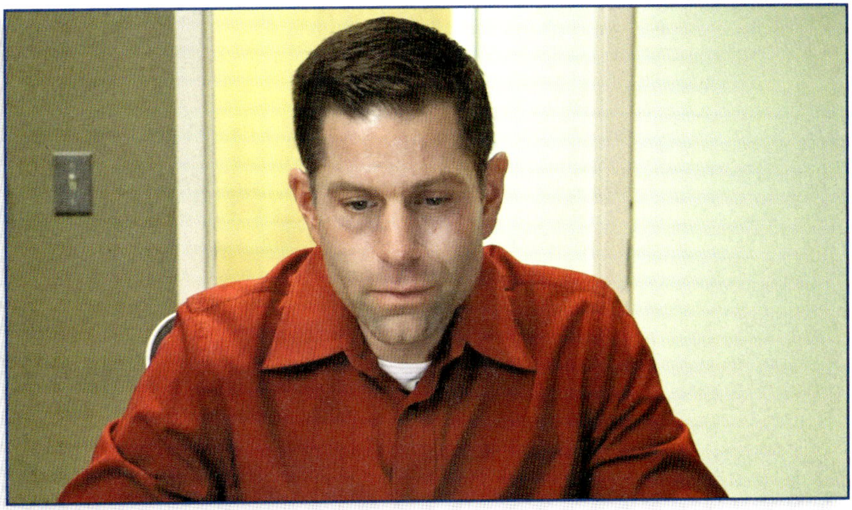

Medical conditions and illnesses can suddenly trigger an unexpected medical emergency. In general, suspect a serious illness when, without warning, a person suddenly appears weak, ill, or in severe pain.

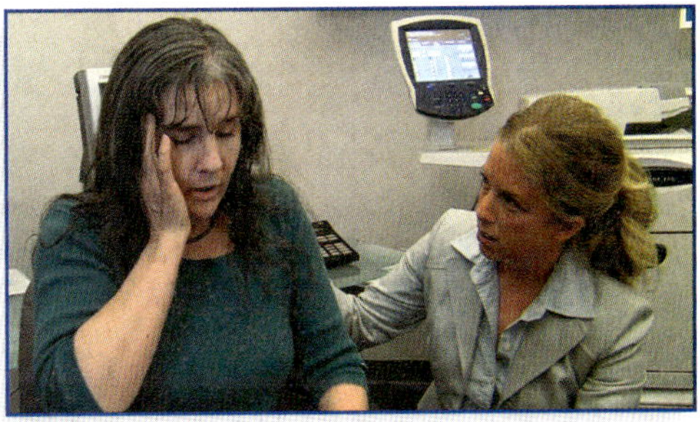

In many cases, the human body displays warning signs to alert us to serious illness. The most common warning signs of serious illness include the following:

- Altered mental status
- Breathing difficulty or shortness of breath
- Pain, severe pressure, or discomfort in the chest

Altered Mental Status

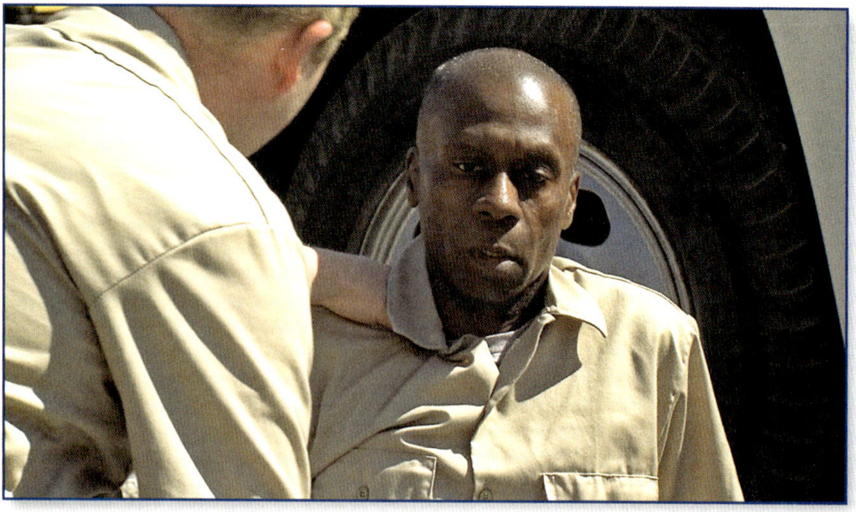

Caused by a number of medical conditions, as well as the use of alcohol, medications, or drugs, an altered mental status is a significant or unusual change in a person's personality, behavior, or consciousness. It is an indication of a change in brain function.

Regardless of the cause, an altered mental status is a warning sign of a serious problem and is considered a medical emergency.

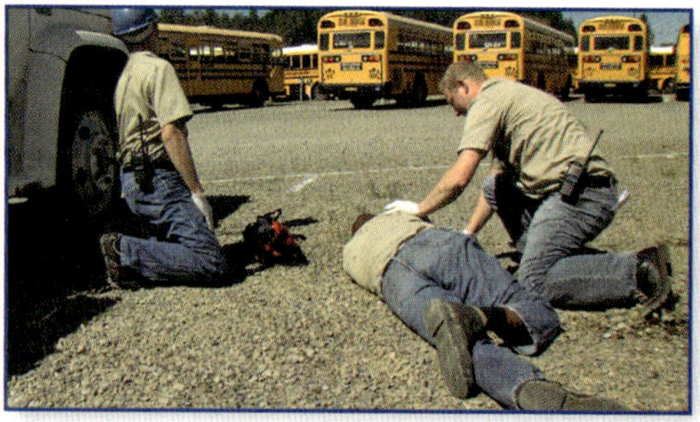

- Activate EMS.
- Position the person for comfort.
- Calm and reassure the person as best you can.
- If responsiveness becomes severely diminished, consider placing in a recovery position to protect the airway.
- Reassess regularly until another provider or EMS personnel take over. The condition could deteriorate quickly and require additional care.

Fainting

Fainting is a momentary loss of consciousness caused by an unexpected drop in blood pressure and blood flow to the brain. Anxiety, fear, pain, stress, standing in place too long, or rapid movements in position, such as standing up quickly from a seated or lying position, can all result in someone feeling faint or fainting. A medication or underlying medical condition might also contribute to the cause.

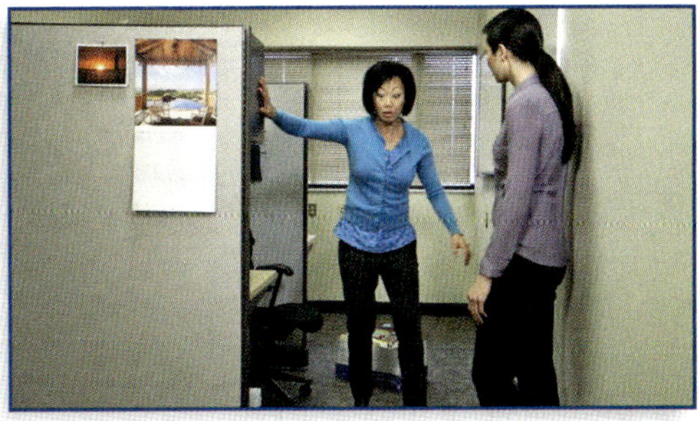

If someone complains of suddenly feeling warm, lightheaded, or that his or her vision is narrowing, follow these guidelines:

- Quickly lay the person flat on his or her back on the ground.
- You can elevate the feet about 6 to 12 inches, which allows blood from the legs to move back into the body.
- Do not elevate the feet if it causes pain or you suspect a person may be injured.

This is a temporary condition that should pass quickly and allow the person to get back to normal activities.

Stroke

A stroke, or brain attack, occurs when the blood supply to a portion of the brain is suddenly interrupted. This most commonly occurs when a blood clot obstructs a blood vessel in the brain. A stroke can also occur when a weak spot in a blood vessel wall, known as an aneurysm, bursts open and bleeds into surrounding brain tissue.

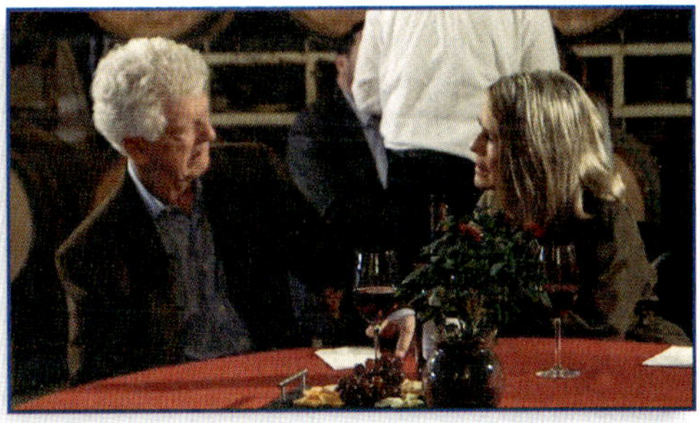

Signs of a stroke can vary depending on where the damage is located. The signs tend to show up suddenly:

- Numbness or weakness of the face, arm, or leg, especially on one side of the body
- Confusion
- A change in the ability to speak or be understood
- Changes in sight and balance
- A severe, sudden headache

Medications are available at hospitals that can limit the severity of a stroke. The earlier they can be given the better.

Early bystander recognition, along with rapid transport to a hospital, is critical for limiting damage, or even for survival.

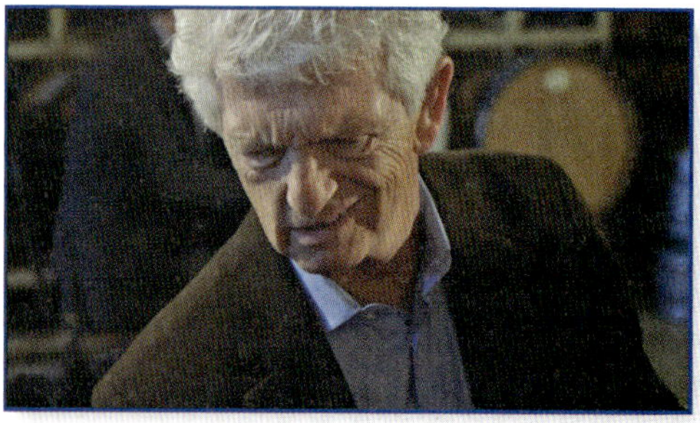

A simple stroke assessment, such as FAST, helps decrease the time it takes to suspect a stroke, activate EMS, and get a person treated in a hospital.

- **F**ace droop: Ask the person to smile. Look to see if the smile is uneven.
- **A**rm drift: Ask the person to raise both arms. Look to see if one drifts back down.
- **S**peech difficulty: Ask the person to speak a simple sentence. Listen for slurring or difficulty.
- **T**ime to activate EMS: If the person has trouble with any of these tasks, activate EMS immediately. Report the time the person was last seen normal to EMS personnel.

Overall, do not give anything to eat or drink. Be prepared for the possibility of sudden cardiac arrest, and the need for CPR and the use of an AED.

A person experiencing a stroke can become frustrated at being unable to move or communicate clearly. The person may appear confused but still be aware of what is happening.

Stay close. Calm, comfort, and reassure the person until another provider or EMS personnel take over.

Hypoglycemia

Diabetes is a disease in which the body cannot effectively use sugar for energy. Hypoglycemia, or low blood sugar, is a diabetic condition that can rapidly develop and become life threatening. Early recognition and treatment by a first aid provider can prevent the condition from worsening.

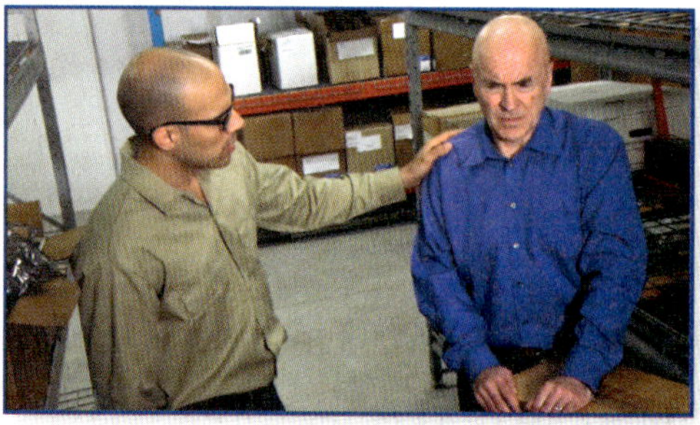

Suspect hypoglycemia with anyone who begins to act oddly or becomes confused. The person may be trembling or shaking, and his or her skin may be pale, cool, and sweaty.

If the person is unable to communicate clearly, look for a medical alert bracelet or necklace which may help identify the underlying condition. You can also check with others about the person's medical history or medications he or she may be taking.

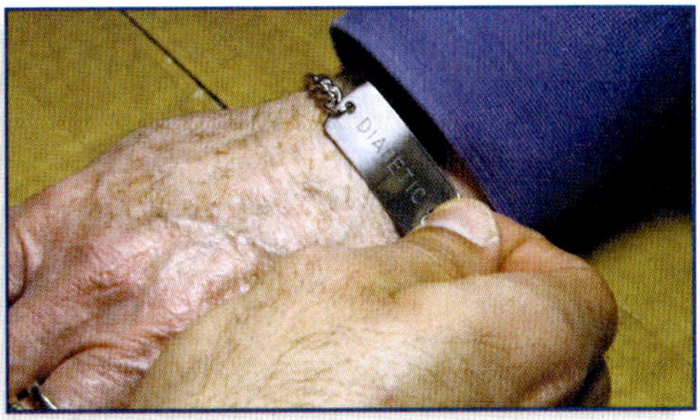

If someone is unresponsive, unable to follow simple commands, or has difficulty swallowing, follow these guidelines:

- Quickly activate EMS.
- Do not give anything to eat or drink.
- Provide any required supportive care.

If the person is responsive and can swallow without difficulty, follow these guidelines:

- Provide about 15 to 20 grams of oral glucose tablets to chew, if they are available.
- If glucose tablets are not available, use something with dietary sugar instead, such as orange juice, candy, fruit leather, or whole milk. Things that use artificial sweeteners will not help.

It is important to note that insulin is not considered an emergency medication. It is never appropriate to administer insulin to a diabetic person in an emergency setting.

Calm, comfort, and reassure the person. If the person responds to the sugar, his or her mental status will gradually improve.

If there is no response to sugar within 10 to 15 minutes or the condition worsens, activate EMS, and provide additional glucose or sugar. Reassess regularly until another provider or EMS personnel take over.

Seizure

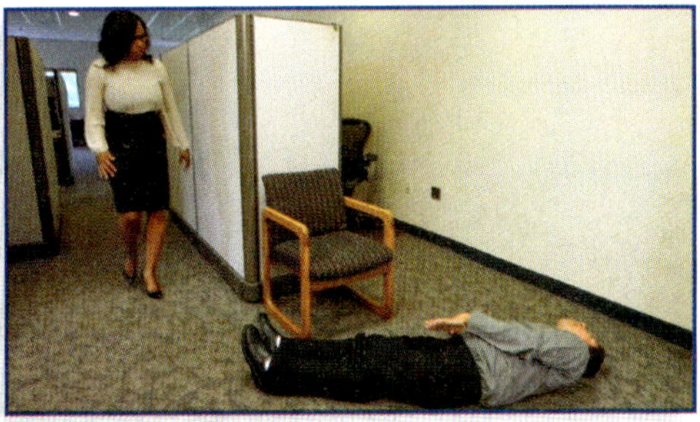

Generalized seizures are triggered by excessive electrical activity within the brain. The result is uncontrolled muscle convulsions throughout the body. Typically, seizures happen without warning. Jerking movements of the body occur and breathing may seem absent. The person can lose control of his or her bowel or bladder, and may vomit.

While there are many things that can cause a seizure to occur, the care provided is always the same:

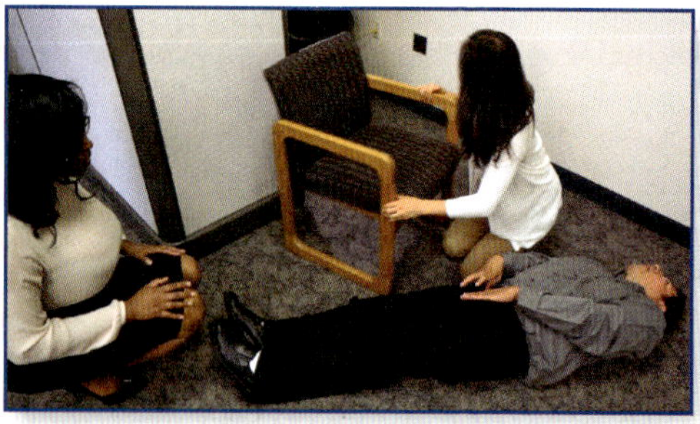

- Protect the person from injury during the seizure.
- Move objects away that he or she may bump into. Protect the person's head from injury as a priority.
- Do not restrain the person. Allow the seizure to take its course.
- If possible, roll the person onto his or her side to allow saliva to drain from his or her mouth.
- Do not put anything in the person's mouth, including your finger. There is no danger of the tongue being swallowed.

Activate EMS if the person does or experiences any of the following:

- Is injured or vomits during the seizure
- Has no history of seizure
- Has multiple seizures or continues to seize for more than 5 minutes

Most seizures last only a short time and stop without any special treatment. Once stopped, place the person in the recovery position to protect the airway. If responsiveness and breathing are absent after a seizure stops, begin CPR and use an AED, if available.

Normally, once a seizure stops, responsiveness improves slowly over time. Provide continual reassurance as the person improves. Provide privacy to minimize embarrassment. it is best to not allow the person to perform actions, such as driving or operating machinery, that could pose a risk for additional injury. Continue to monitor until EMS personnel take over care or the person returns to normal.

Knowledge Check

Often with an altered mental status, a person may develop a severely diminished level of responsiveness. What can you do to help that person to protect and maintain an open airway?

Breathing Difficulty, Shortness of Breath

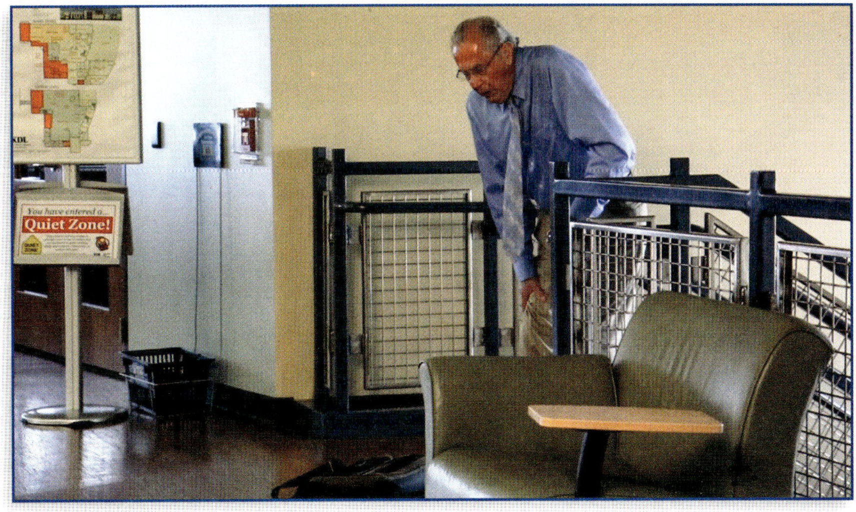

Breathing difficulty or shortness of breath is a medical emergency. It is generally caused by an underlying medical illness such as asthma, allergic reaction, heart failure, or lung disease.

At rest, normal breathing is regular and effortless. You may first suspect difficulty when there is a noticeable increase in the effort to breathe and the rate at which breaths are occurring. Coughing, wheezing, or other unusual breathing sounds may occur.

A bluish purple tissue color, especially in the lips or fingers, indicates a developing lack of oxygen and is a serious warning sign.

- Do not wait to see if condition will improve. Activate EMS without delay.
- If an AED is available, have someone get it.
- Allow the person to find the most comfortable position in which to breathe.
- Loosen any tight clothing.
- Breathing difficulty can quickly become life threatening. Be prepared to provide CPR and attach an AED if breathing stops.
- Reassess regularly until another provider or EMS take over.

Asthma and Inhalers

Asthma is a medical condition in which certain things can trigger a physical reaction in the lungs and make it difficult for a person to breathe.

Quick-relief medications, delivered with an inhaler device, work fast to help control asthma symptoms. If the person has a prescribed inhaler assist him or her in using it. Activate EMS immediately if the symptoms seem serious, gets worse, or if there is no response to the medication within 5 minutes.

Severe Allergic Reaction

A severe allergic reaction, known as anaphylaxis, is an extreme response of the body's immune system to something it is sensitive to. There are common things that can initiate a severe reaction:

- Bee stings
- Peanuts
- Latex
- Penicillin

When anaphylaxis occurs, the airway can become constricted due to swelling of the throat, making it difficult to breathe. Wheezing may be heard. Other symptoms may include the following:

- Swelling of the lips, eyelids, and face
- Itchy raised lumps, or hives, on the face and chest
- Nausea and abdominal cramping

A severe allergic reaction can develop rapidly. In general, the faster the reaction occurs, the more severe it is. Without treatment, death can occur within a few minutes.[4]

When assisting someone during an allergic reaction, follow these guidelines:

- Allow the person to find the most comfortable position in which to breathe.
- A person with a history of allergic reactions may carry a prescribed epinephrine auto-injector. Epinephrine can quickly reverse the effects of the reaction and may be life-saving.
- Auto-injectors use a spring-loaded needle to rapidly administer a measured, single dose of epinephrine. They are easy to use with minimal training. If the person has an auto-injector available, assist him or her in self-administering it.
- Activate EMS. If you are able, do it while the auto-injector is being used.
- If the person has not responded to an initial dose of epinephrine and EMS is still at least 5 to 10 minutes away, a second dose may be given.
- Reassess regularly until another provider or EMS personnel take over.

ASSISTING WITH MEDICATION

State laws and regulations may prescribe specific practices, rules, and standards for administering prescribed medication to another person. Be aware of the regulations in your local area.

Knowledge Check

You have responded as a first aid provider to a coworker who is having difficulty breathing. You suspect an underlying medical condition is the cause and the person does not have his prescribed inhaler. While waiting for EMS to arrive, you see his condition has gotten much worse. He looks exhausted. What is your greatest concern at this point and how have you prepared to deal with it?

Pain, Severe Pressure, or Discomfort in the Chest

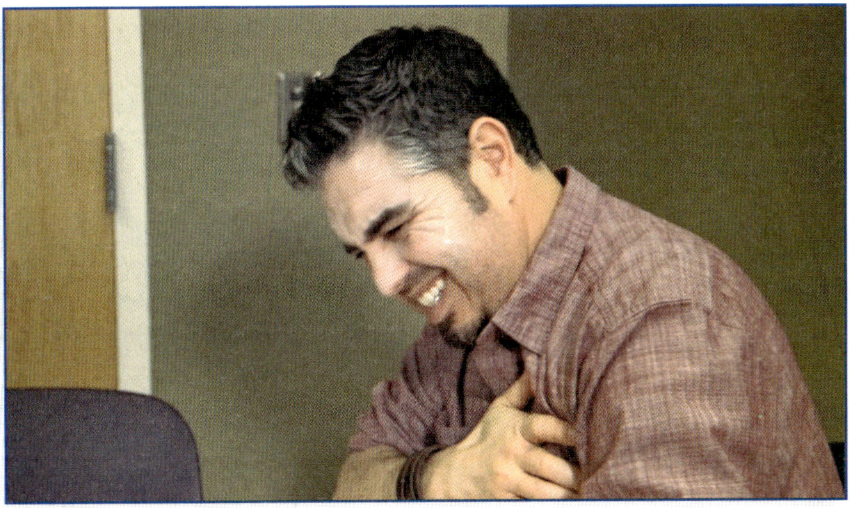

Acute coronary syndrome (ACS) occurs when there is reduced blood flow to the tissues of the heart. Often described as a heart attack, ACS is a serious condition that can result in significant damage to the heart.

Someone with ACS will generally experience pain, pressure, or discomfort in the chest, although women often do not experience chest pain and may describe indigestion, weakness, or fatigue. Shortness of breath, nausea, and lightheadedness can also occur. The person may experience pain in the arms or back. The person's skin may become pale, cool, and sweaty.

A person who has had previous heart problems is at risk for reoccurrence. Ask the person or any bystanders about prior problems, or medications being taken.

If you suspect a heart-related problem, do not try to transport the person to a hospital yourself. Activate EMS immediately, even if the person does not want you to. While waiting for EMS to arrive, follow these guidelines:

- If an AED is available, have someone get it so that it's nearby if needed.
- Allow the person to find the most comfortable position in which to breathe.
- Loosen tight clothing.
- Calm, comfort, and reassure the person.

- A person who is having a heart attack may deny it. This is a common occurrence in this situation. Accept it, but never let this alter your approach to care.
- The early administration of aspirin can be life-saving for a person having a heart attack. Encourage the person to chew and swallow 1 adult (325 mg), or 2 to 4 low-dose (81 mg) "baby" aspirin.

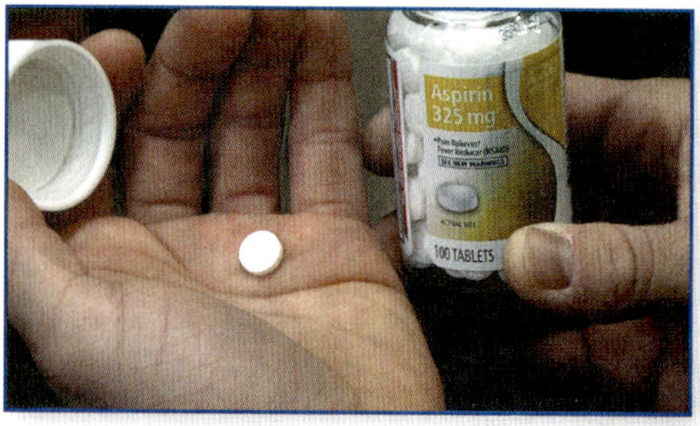

- Do not encourage aspirin use if the person has an allergy to aspirin, evidence of a stroke, a recent bleeding problem, the pain does not appear to be related to the heart, or if you are uncertain or uncomfortable with giving the aspirin.
- Someone with a heart condition may carry a prescribed medication known as nitroglycerin. If so, assist the person in the self-administration of it.

Whenever a heart attack is suspected, be prepared for the possibility of sudden cardiac arrest, and the need for CPR and the use of an AED. Continue to reassure the person until another provider or EMS personnel take over.

Heart Disease

Heart disease, through heart attacks and strokes, is the leading cause of death for men and women in the United States. Statistics indicate more than 1 in 4 deaths was related to heart disease; half of the deaths were women.

A healthy lifestyle can lower the risk of heart disease:

- Follow a healthy diet to prevent or reduce high blood pressure and high blood cholesterol
- Maintain a healthy weight
- Control alcohol intake
- Don't smoke
- Exercise regularly

Knowledge Check

True or false? A person who is having a heart attack may deny it.

Poisoning

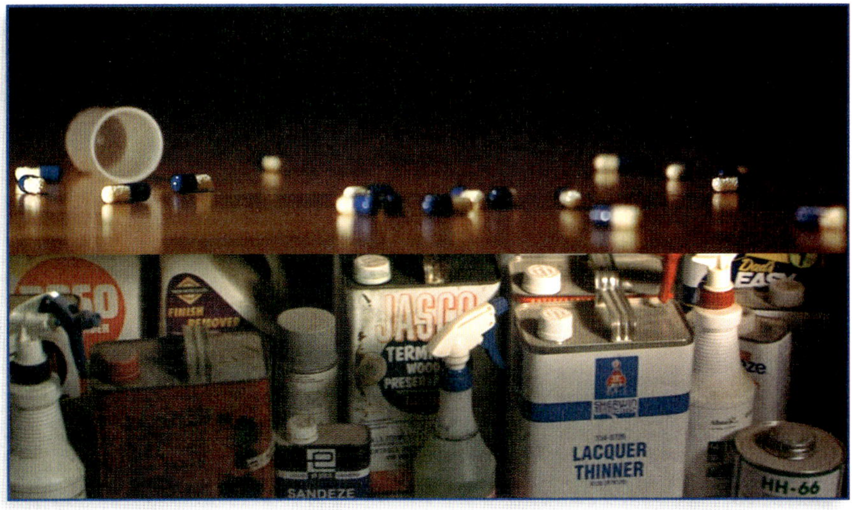

Any substance that can enter the body and create a harmful reaction in the body can be described as a poison.

Ingested Poisoning

By far, poisoning most often occurs by ingestion. Children under 6 years account for over half of all poisonings. Most poisoning deaths are accidental, but some deaths are intentional.

Common ingested poisons include the following:

- Prescribed medications
- Personal care products
- Household cleaning products

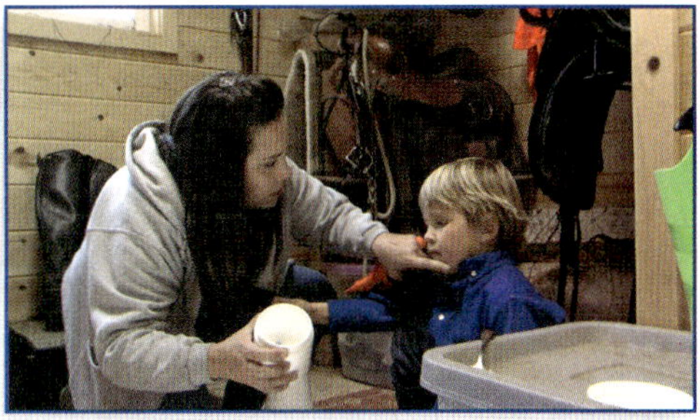

The effects of ingested poisons are wide ranging and often resemble those of common illnesses. These are symptoms that may occur:

- Abdominal pain or cramping
- Nausea
- Vomiting
- Altered mental status

Often, the ingestion is described by the person. Open and empty containers, unusual smells, and odd staining on clothes, skin, or lips may be present.

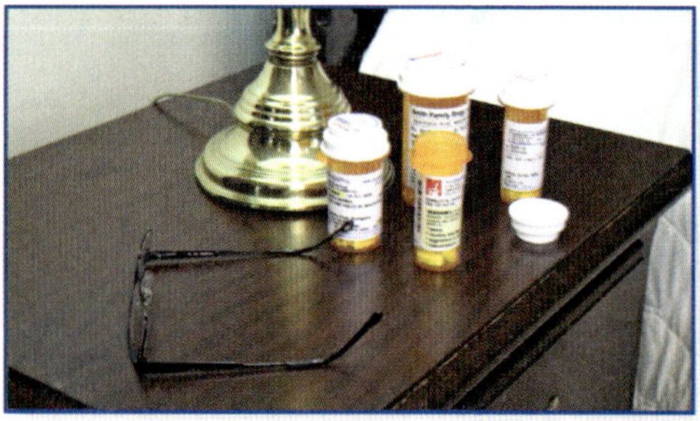

If you suspect a person has ingested something poisonous, act quickly. Activate EMS if the person is displaying any serious signs or symptoms.

In the United States, calling the national Poison Help line at 1-800-222-1222 automatically transfers you to a regional poison control center. Poison control centers can quickly provide information regarding the immediate treatment to exposure to any substance.[5]

You can help EMS providers and the poison control center by clearly identifying the substance and providing details about the incident. Save any vomit, bottles, or containers for EMS. While waiting for help to arrive, follow these guidelines:

- Do not administer anything by mouth for any poison ingestion unless advised to do so by a poison control center or EMS personnel.
- Keep the person still.
- Calm, comfort, and reassure.
- Reassess the person regularly until another first aid provider or EMS personnel take over.

Inhaled Poisoning

Inhaled poisoning occurs when a harmful substance is breathed in. Common inhaled poisons include carbon monoxide, natural gas, solvent fumes, and chemical vapors.

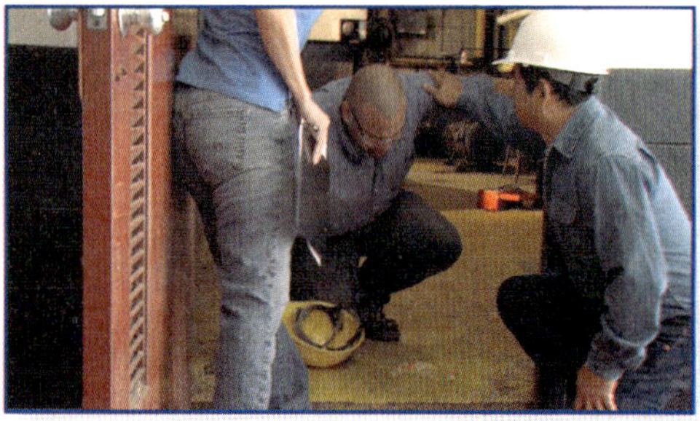

Symptoms of inhaled poisoning may include the following:

- Headache
- Nausea
- Dizziness
- Difficulty breathing
- Altered mental status

Some poisons, such as natural gas, have a telltale odor. Other poisons, such as carbon monoxide, do not. Suspect inhaled poisoning whenever someone is working in an enclosed space and he or she is feeling ill.

Make sure it is safe for you to help, and then follow these guidelines when assisting someone who is suffering from inhaled poisoning:

- If you can do so without risk to yourself, immediately move the person to fresh air.
- Help the person to find a comfortable position.
- Activate EMS if the person is displaying any serious signs or symptoms.
- Call the national Poison Help line at 1-800-222-1222 for additional directions on care. Help identify the substance and provide details about the incident.
- Reassess regularly until another first aid provider or EMS personnel take over.

Poisonous Plants

Direct skin contact with plants such as poison oak, poison sumac, and poison ivy can cause problematic skin reactions. Usually occurring within hours or days of exposure, these reactions result in itchy, red skin rashes with open sores.

If you have been exposed, you may be able to prevent a reaction by washing the affected area with soap and water as soon as possible to remove the oily plant resin. Carefully handle and wash any clothes or tools that may have been exposed.

If a minor reaction occurs, commercial relief products are available to ease symptoms. Seek medical attention if the reaction seems serious.

Alcohol, Drugs, and Medications

The use, or overuse, of alcohol, drugs, or medications can result in serious life-threatening problems. A diminished mental status can result in the loss of an airway. Breathing can become depressed and stop. Vomiting can occur.

In quantity, these things can become toxic or poisonous and result in internal damage to body organs and functions. Treat as with any other suspected ingested poisoning. Call the Poison Help line at 1-800-222-1222 for treatment recommendations.

Knowledge Check

In the United States, calling the national Poison Help line automatically transfers you to a regional poison control center. Poison control centers can quickly provide information regarding the immediate treatment to exposure of any substance. What is the number to call?

Severe Abdominal Pain

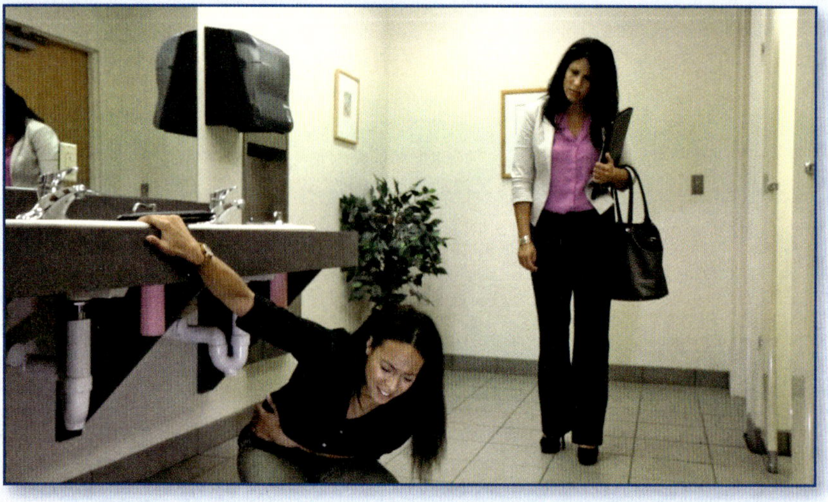

Severe abdominal pain may be a warning sign of serious illness, especially if it appears suddenly or is a new experience for the person. There are many important organs in the abdomen. A wide variety of problems could occur and result in intense pain. Without a professional medical assessment, it is impossible to accurately determine what the underlying cause is.

Early suspicion and rapid transport to a hospital may help to prevent the development of a life-threatening condition. The abdomen may be rigid or tender to the touch. The person may become nauseated and vomit. If a person's symptoms seem severe, or you are not sure, follow these guidelines:

- Activate EMS without delay.
- A person complaining of severe abdominal pain will typically try to find a position of comfort, often with the knees raised, to relieve the pain. Help the person to maintain this position.
- Provide calming reassurance until EMS personnel take over.

Internal bleeding related to a pregnancy is one cause of abdominal pain. Light, irregular discharge of blood through the vagina, or spotting, is normal in a pregnancy. However, significant bleeding, especially late in the pregnancy, is a serious medical emergency. Severe abdominal cramping and pain can occur. Her skin may become cool, sweaty, and pale in color. She may be weak and lightheaded.

If a pregnant woman is experiencing symptoms like these, do the following:

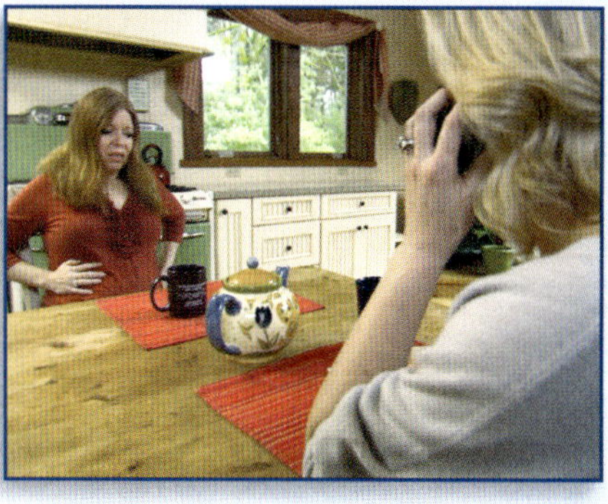

- Activate EMS immediately.
- When lying face up, the baby puts pressure on the main vein that returns blood to the heart. Lay the mother on her left side to improve blood flow to both the mother and baby.
- Have her place a sanitary pad over the vaginal opening. Do not insert anything inside the vagina.
- Treat for shock. Help maintain a normal body temperature.
- Do not give anything to eat or drink.
- Calm, comfort, and reassure her.
- Reassess regularly until EMS personnel take over.

Knowledge Check

You respond as a trained first aid provider to a sales clerk in the store where you work. You find the 25-year-old woman curled up on a couch in the break room, complaining of a severe stabbing pain in her abdomen. As you provide care, what considerations should you take about positioning her to help relieve the pain?

Heat Emergencies

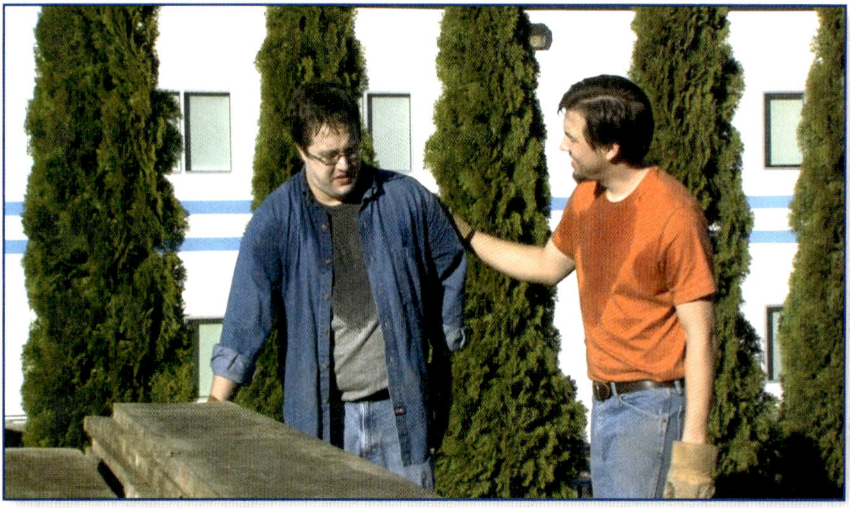

Heat-related problems occur when a body's normal temperature-reducing mechanisms get overwhelmed and become inefficient or stop working. This is especially true during vigorous physical activity.[6]

Heat Exhaustion

When a person is exposed to warm, humid temperatures, his or her internal body temperature begins to rise. Normally, the body reacts by sweating, which evaporates and pulls heat out and away from the body.

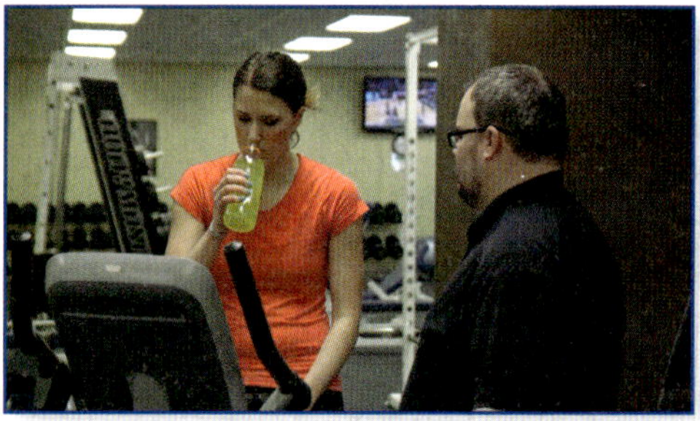

Simply rehydrating someone suspected of being dehydrated due to physical exertion and sweating could prevent serious heat-related problems from developing. Drinking a carbohydrate-electrolyte drink, such as a sports drink, works well to do this. Use water if a sports drink is not available. Coconut water and 2% milk have also shown to promote rehydration after exertion. Lemon tea-based drinks and Chinese tea with caffeine have a comparable rehydration effect to water.

Heat exhaustion can occur as a combined result of a rising internal temperature and dehydration.

Signs of heat exhaustion include the following:

- Heavy sweating
- Pale, cool, sweaty skin
- Nausea and vomiting
- Headache
- Dizziness
- Feeling weak

Although it may not appear serious, treat heat exhaustion quickly. Without early recognition and treatment, it could progress to heat stroke, a life-threatening condition.

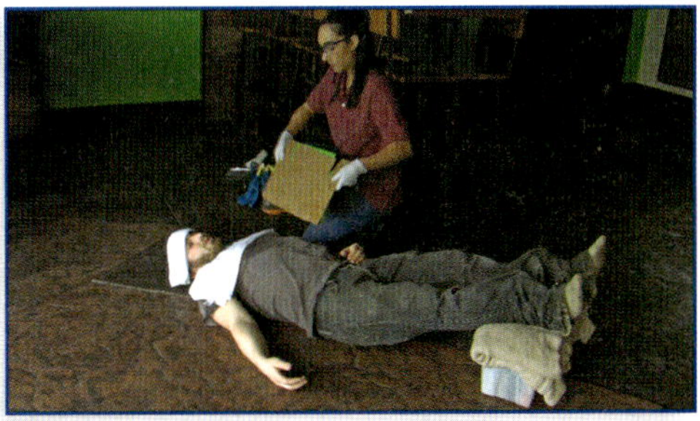

- Have the person stop any activity and move him or her to a cooler place.
- Loosen or remove excess clothing.
- Have the person lie down. If the person is uninjured, consider raising his or her legs 6 to 12 inches. Do not elevate the legs if it causes pain or the person is injured.
- Spray water on or apply cool, wet cloths to the head and torso. Use a fan to increase the cooling effect.
- If the person is able to follow simple commands and swallow without trouble, encourage the person to drink fluids, preferably a carbohydrate-electrolyte sports drink. Use water if a sports drink is not available. Do not give anything to drink if the person is confused or he or she has difficulty swallowing.

In most cases, the person's condition will gradually get better. If the person does not improve or seems to get worse, activate EMS.

Heat Cramps

Heat cramps are uncontrollable muscle spasms that can affect the calves, arms, abdominal muscles, and back. They can occur suddenly and be very painful.

Stretching and direct pressure to the cramping muscle may help. Delay further activity until the cramping has been resolved.

Heat Stroke

Heat stroke is a condition in which body temperature rises because the body's normal cooling systems are overwhelmed, or simply shut down as a result of extended exposure to a hot environment. It is a serious medical emergency and can quickly cause permanent damage to the brain.

- The person will be very warm, even hot to the touch.
- Heavy sweating could be present, but in many cases the skin can be red and completely dry.
- Typically, the person will be confused and could have trouble communicating.
- The person may become unresponsive and could experience a seizure.

Activate EMS immediately. The most important action a first aid provider can take is to begin immediate cooling with the resources available:

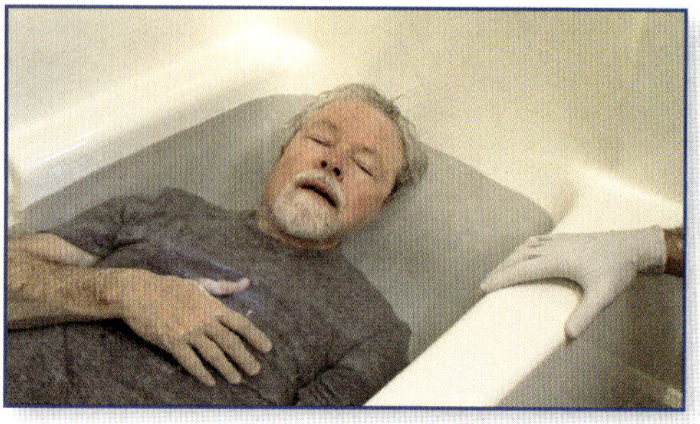

- When possible, the best method for cooling is to immerse the person up to the chin in cold water.
- If immersion is not possible, spray or pour cold water on the person, and fan him or her to increase cooling effect.
- Apply cold packs to the neck, groin, and armpits.
- Cover the person with a cold, wet sheet, and use a fan to enhance cooling.
- Provide continuous cooling until EMS personnel take over care.

With early recognition and effective cooling, most people suffering from heat stroke will survive.

Knowledge Check

You are volunteering as a first aid provider at your city's annual 10K run. Most runners have finished but a few are still trickling in. You see in the distance a runner being helped to walk, when he suddenly falls to his knees. You grab your first aid bag and run out to see if you can help. Your primary assessment shows he is very confused. His skin is sweaty, but surprisingly hot to your touch. What should you do for him?

Cold Emergencies

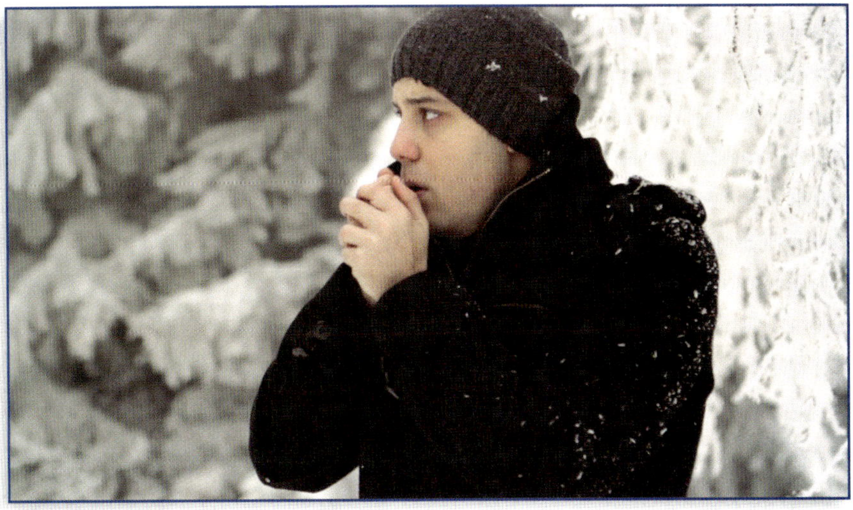

A cold or cool, wet environment can result in a lowering of internal body temperature. Hypothermia and frostbite are the most dangerous cold-related conditions.

Hypothermia

Hypothermia, a generalized cooling of the body, occurs when the internal core body temperature has decreased to 95° F or less. It can be a life-threatening condition.

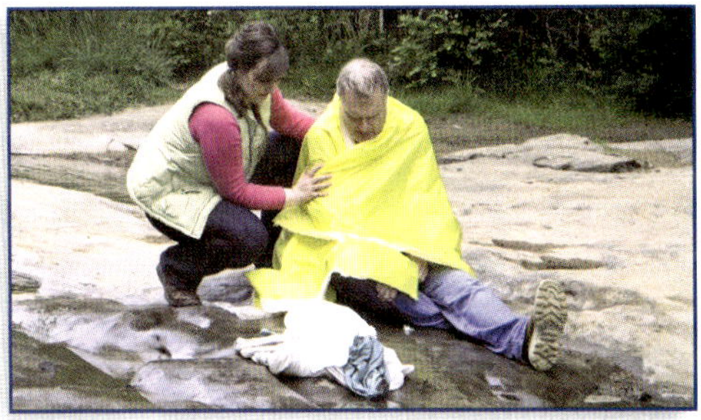

Look for early signs of hypothermia, such as the following:

- Pale, cold skin
- Uncontrollable shivering
- Loss of coordination

As hypothermia progresses, shivering may stop. Breathing and heart rate slow down. Body processes can become impaired and may fail.

- Remove wet clothing and cover person with something warm and dry.
- Activate EMS.
- Cardiac arrest could occur. Get an AED if one is accessible.
- To care for the person, move him or her to a warmer place. Move the person slowly and without rapid movements.
- Cover the head and neck to retain body heat.

If you are far from professional medical care, begin actively rewarming the person. Place him or her near a heat source. Put containers of warm, but not hot, water in contact with the person's skin.

It is best to recognize and treat hypothermia early. The chance for survival decreases as the condition progresses.

Frostbite

Frostbite occurs when skin and underlying body tissue freezes. Body parts that are commonly exposed to extreme cold, such as the fingers, toes, earlobes, cheeks, and nose, are the most likely to be affected.

Lowering tissue temperature, prior to freezing, may cause a pins-and-needles sensation and throbbing.

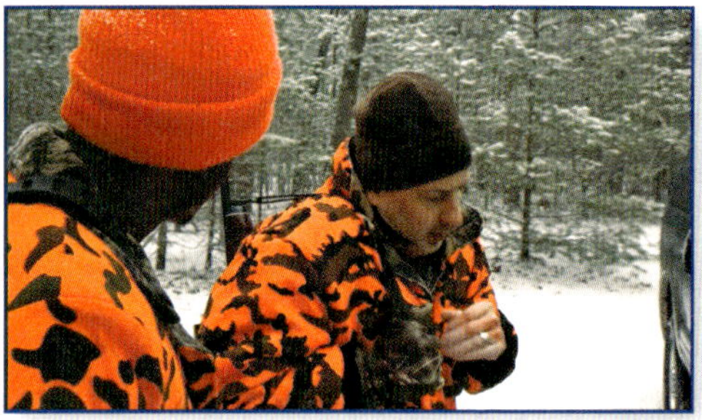

Freezing could be prevented by using a simple skin-to-skin rewarming technique, such as holding the affected part in a warm hand.

Signs of freezing include a loss of feeling in the affected part and firm, pale, cold, numb skin.

If you suspect frostbite, quickly get the person to a warmer place. When EMS is close, or there is any chance that the part may refreeze, do not try to rewarm the frostbitten area.

- Remove any wet clothing.
- Do not rub or massage the affected area or disturb blisters on frostbitten skin.
- Remove all jewelry from the affected areas.
- Place clean pads between frostbitten fingers and toes.
- Wrap the affected part with a clean towel or pad.
- Keep the affected part still and protected. Provide ongoing reassurance until EMS providers can take over care.

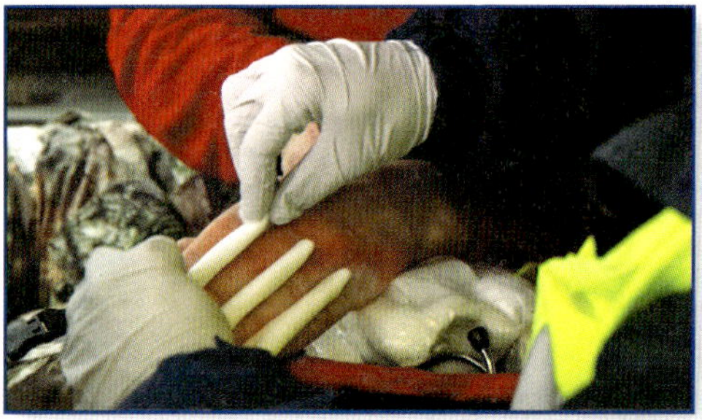

If you are far from professional medical care, and there is no chance refreezing will occur, rewarm the affected part yourself:

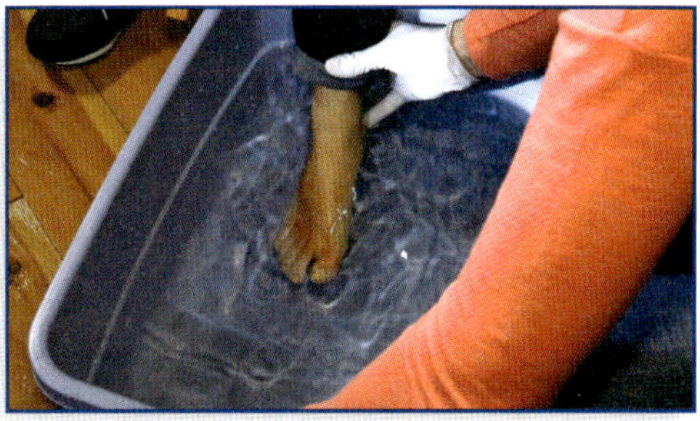

- Immerse the frostbitten area in warm water for 20 to 30 minutes. The water should be warm, not hot – just above normal body temperature.
- Check and maintain the water temperature often.
- Severe burning pain, swelling, blistering, and color changes may occur.

Chemical warmers can reach temperatures that result in burns. They should not be used to rewarm frostbitten tissue.

Do not let the person use the affected part after it is thawed. Get him or her to professional medical care as soon as you are able.

Knowledge Check

You are trying to wrap up some repairs at an outside job site with another electrician. It has been a miserable rainy day and the temperature is going down late in the day. Your partner did not prepare as well as you did for the cold, rainy conditions and his light cotton clothes have been completely soaked through. You look up at him from a repair you have been concentrating on. It looks like he is having trouble grasping his pliers and is visibly shivering. You ask him if he is okay and he has trouble responding to you. What do you suspect may be occurring?

Stinging Insects

Many insects such as bees, wasps, and fire ants may sting when agitated or in defense of their nests or territories.

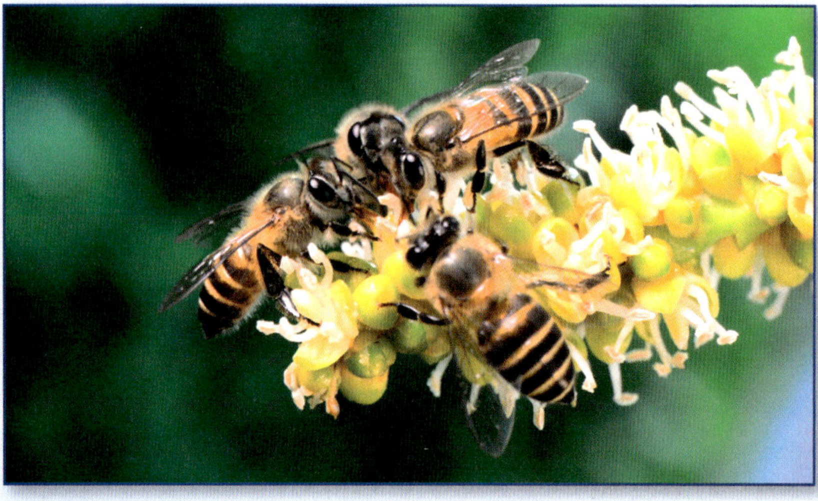

While wasps and fire ants can sting repeatedly, the stinger of a honey bee detaches from its body, remains embedded in the skin, and continues to inject venom.

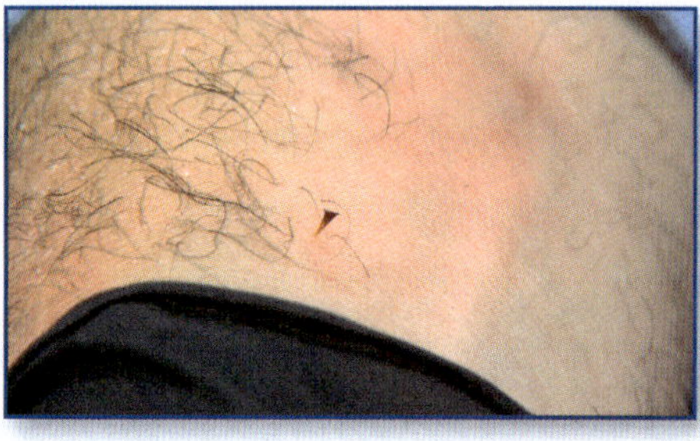

- If a stinger is present in the skin, remove it as quickly as possible.
- Local pain, redness, swelling, and itching generally occur at the sting site.
- In general, care for bites and stings by washing the site with soap and water.
- As a precaution for swelling, always remove jewelry from the affected area.
- Cover the area with an adhesive bandage or a pad.
- Use local cooling to help reduce swelling and pain.

It is possible for a life-threatening allergic reaction to develop. Monitor for at least 30 minutes to see if condition worsens.

If you think someone is developing a severe allergic reaction, immediately activate EMS. If the person affected has an epinephrine auto-injector available, assist the person in self-administration.

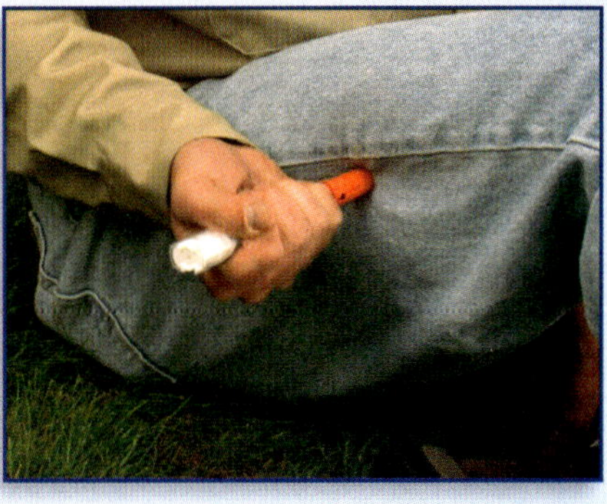

Additional Information

Infectious diseases can be transmitted through insect stings. The latest information on this can be found by visiting the U.S. Centers for Disease Control and Prevention website at www.cdc.gov.

Knowledge Check

You and a coworker are outdoors at lunch when she suddenly shouts that something stung her. You look at her forearm and see a stinger that is still embedded in her skin. What should you do?

Snakebites

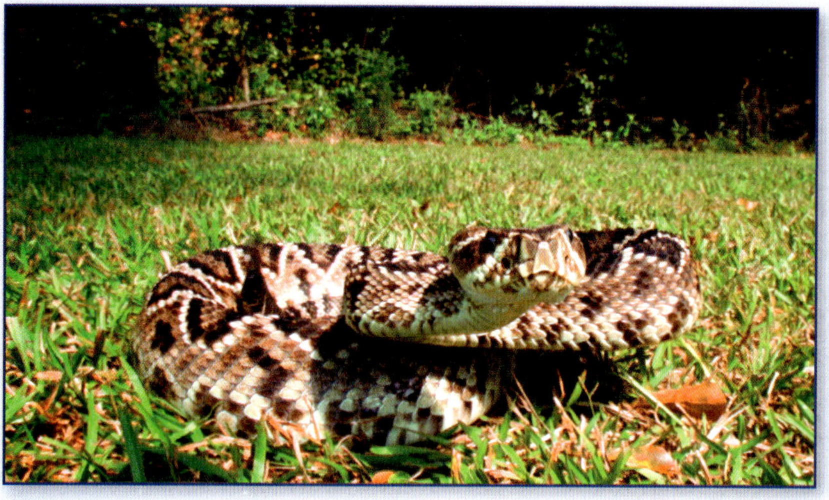

Only a few types of venomous snakes are found in North America. Very few of the snakebites that occur are fatal. However, because fatalities have occurred, a suspected venomous snakebite should be considered and treated as a medical emergency.[7]

Pit Viper

Venomous cottonmouths, copperheads, and rattlesnakes are known as pit vipers. Pit vipers strike once and leave a characteristic bite with single or double fang mark. Pit viper bites can cause intense, burning pain and rapid local swelling.

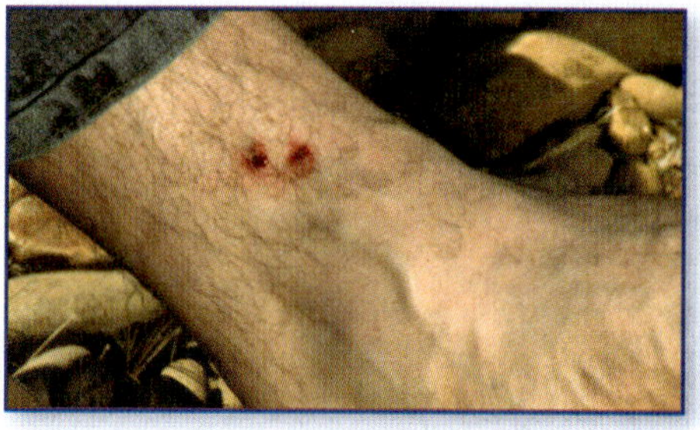

If you suspect a pit viper bite, reassure the person that effective medical treatment is available.

- Have the person sit still and stay calm to slow the spread of venom within the body.
- Activate EMS.
- Remove any rings, or other constricting items from the affected limb.
- Control any bleeding with a clean pad and direct pressure.
- Immobilize the injured part and keep it below heart level.

- Do not apply a tourniquet, cold compresses, or try to suck out the venom by mouth.
- Keep the person warm, reassured, and quiet until EMS providers can take over.

Coral Snake

A venomous coral snake bite differs from that of a pit viper. Instead of a single strike, coral snakes will chew with fixed fangs.

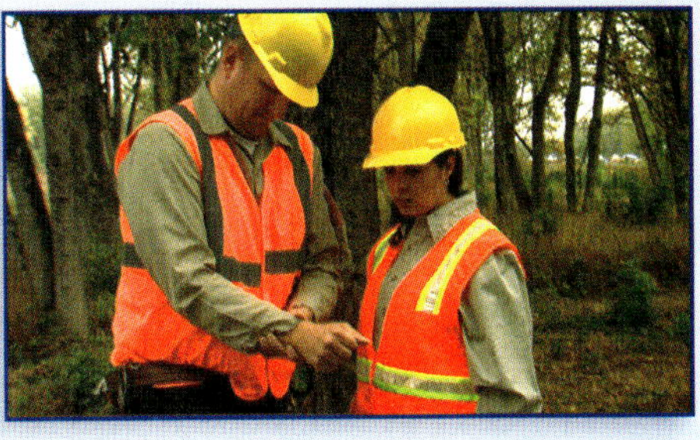

Pain and swelling at the bite site may be minimal or absent. Serious effects are often delayed. When they do appear, symptoms can include the following:

- Abdominal pain
- Nausea and vomiting
- Rapid heartbeat
- Difficulty breathing
- Drooling
- Altered mental status

If you suspect a coral snake bite, have the person sit still and remain calm.

- Activate EMS.
- To slow the spread of venom, apply a pressure bandage around the entire length of the bitten extremity. Wrap toward the body. The bandage should be snug, but not so tight that you can't slip a finger under it.
- Immobilize the injured part and keep it below heart level.
- As with pit vipers, do not apply local cooling.
- Do not try to suck out the venom or use a tourniquet. These treatments are not effective and may be harmful.
- Keep the person warm, reassured, and quiet while awaiting EMS. Move the person only if needed.

Knowledge Check

You and a coworker are doing landscape maintenance when he shouts and scrambles out from behind some bushes. He says he was bitten by a snake and shows you his calf, which appears to have has a double fang mark on it. What type of snake do you suspect was involved?

Spider Bites

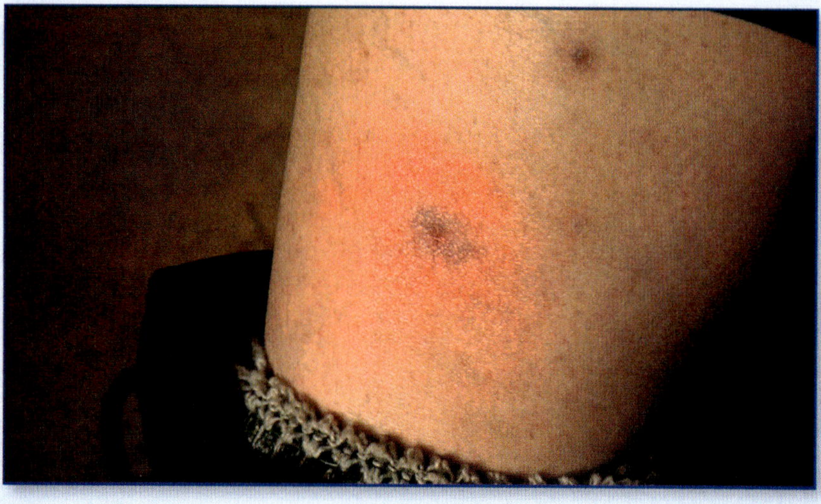

Spiders typically inhabit out-of-the-way places such as wood piles or out buildings. There are certain spiders that can be dangerous to humans; these include the black widow and the brown recluse.

Initially, venomous spider bites are often difficult to identify.

- Small puncture marks and bleeding may be seen.
- Tenderness, swelling, pain, itchiness, and redness at the bite site can develop.
- Over time, cramping pain and muscular rigidity in the body may occur.
- A person may experience fever, weakness, nausea and vomiting, or difficulty breathing.

If you suspect a severe reaction from a spider bite, activate EMS. Keep the person warm, reassured, and quiet while awaiting EMS.

Knowledge Check

You are working with another contractor in an old storage shed when he reacts to a sudden burning sensation on his leg. Due to the dim light, you cannot see anything. When you get outside, there is a small red mark that itches but does not worry him. If he was bitten by a poisonous spider, what may happen?

Tick Bites

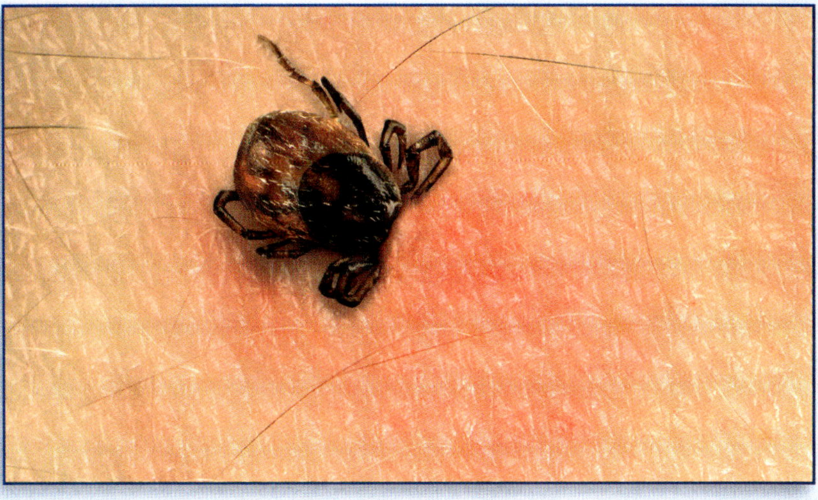

Ticks are blood-feeding insects that are typically found in tall grass and shrubs. When a tick bites, it attaches itself firmly to the skin. The biggest concern with tick bites is the exposure and transmission of infectious disease, most notably Lyme disease.

- To remove an embedded tick, grasp it close to the skin with tweezers or a tick removal tool.
- Pull straight up with a steady, slow motion.
- After removal, clean the area well with soap and water or a disinfecting wipe. When finished, thoroughly wash your hands.

If portions of the tick remain in the skin or you develop a rash or flu-like symptoms, seek further medical attention.

Do not use fingernail polish, petroleum jelly, a glowing hot match, or alcohol to remove a tick. These actions have no proven value and may cause additional problems.

Knowledge Check

What is the biggest concern with a tick bite?

Marine Animal Stings

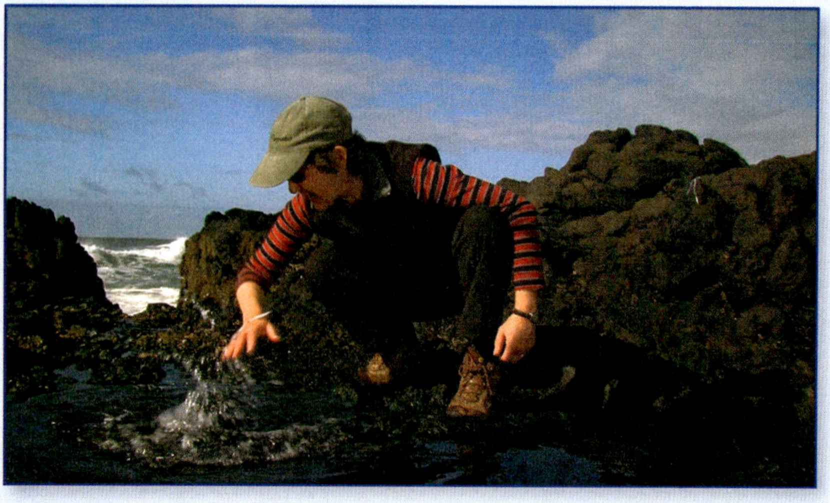

Stings from marine animals, such as fire coral, sea anemones, and jellyfish, can occur when a person is in or around the ocean environment.

Jellyfish

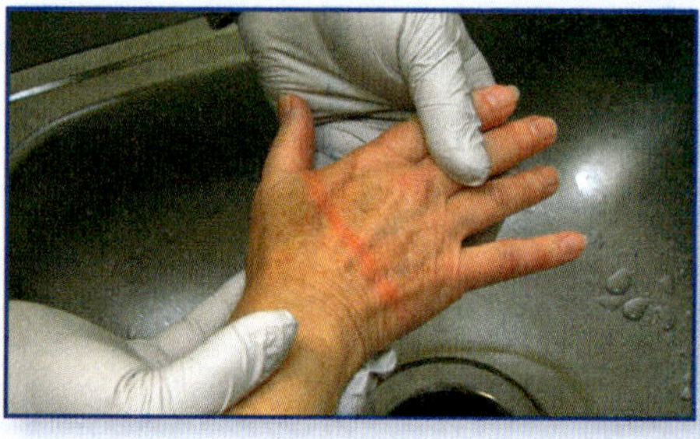

Stings can result in significant pain at the sting site and a raised, red, itchy rash. Wash the sting site liberally with household vinegar as soon as possible for at least 30 seconds to deactivate the venom and prevent further stinging.

To help reduce pain, shower or immerse the sting site with hot water for at least 20 minutes or until the pain subsides. The water should be as hot as the person can safely tolerate.

Stingray

A stingray is a marine animal with a slender tail and venom-filled spines that can puncture the skin and inject venom.

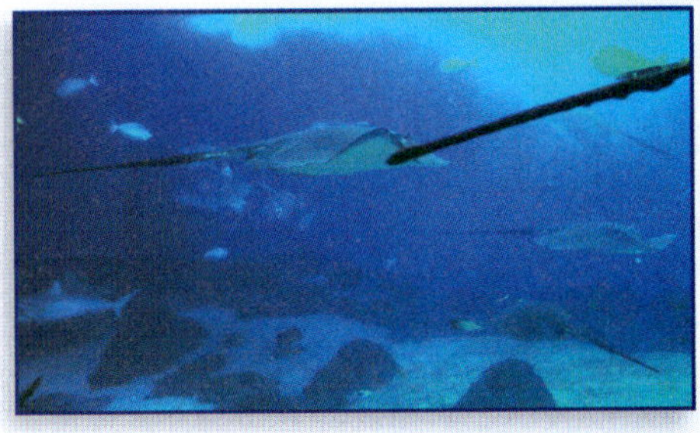

Intense pain can occur at the sting site. Immerse the injured area in water as hot as the person can tolerate for 30 to 90 minutes to deactivate the venom and help relieve pain. Carefully clean out the wound site.

Severe reactions to marine animal stings can include difficulty breathing, heart palpitations, weakness, and fainting. If this occurs, activate EMS immediately. Monitor closely and be prepared to quickly provide supportive care until EMS personnel take over.

Knowledge Check

You are collecting water samples in a tide pool with a coworker when she reaches her hand into the pool and is stung by a jellyfish. What two treatment techniques will help to prevent and relieve pain at the sting site?

Animal and Human Bites

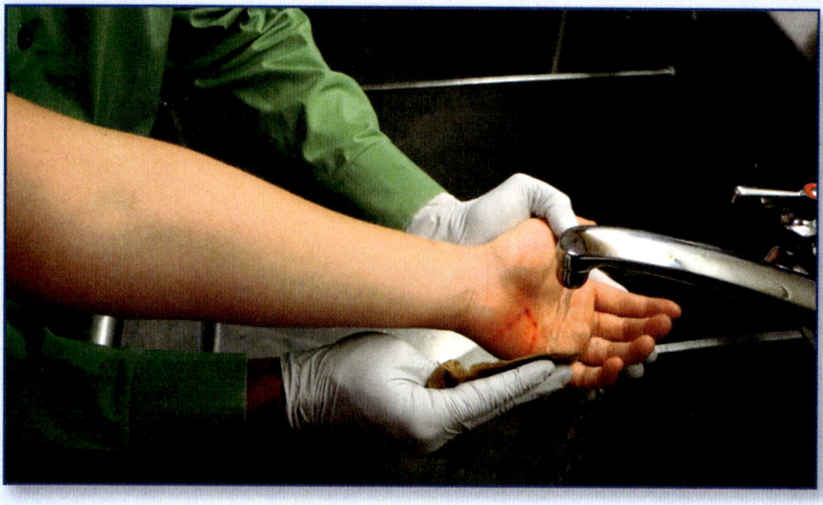

Animal bites can cause significant injury and bacterial infection. Human bites are also of concern.

Bites from animals such as raccoons, skunks, bats, and foxes can also cause rabies. Left untreated, rabies is fatal.

- Control any bleeding with direct pressure.
- Wash the bite and flush with large amounts of water.
- Due to the chance of infection, any animal or human bite that breaks the skin should be evaluated by a medical professional.

Knowledge Check

What is the main concern related to bites from animals like raccoons, skunks, bats, and foxes?

Emotional Considerations

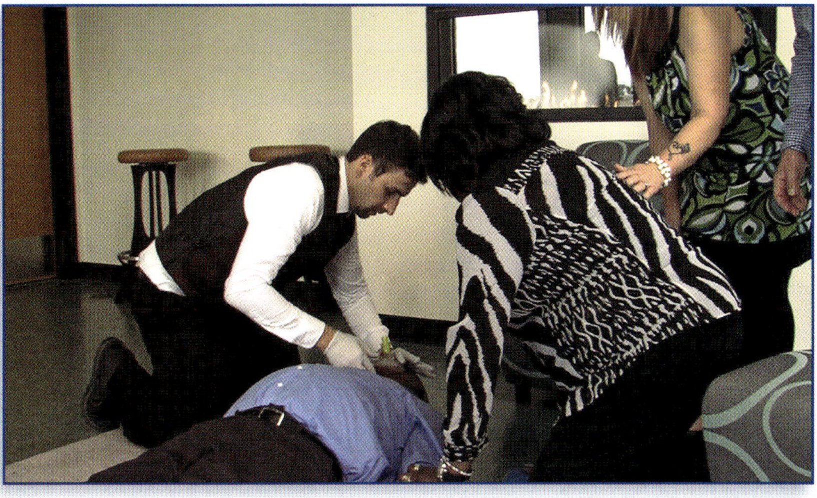

Caring for someone in an emergency can create emotional distress. Exposure to an extreme situation or having a close relationship with those involved can intensify these feelings.

Common reactions include the following:

- Anxiety
- Trembling or shaking
- Sweating
- Nausea
- Fast breathing
- Pounding heartbeat

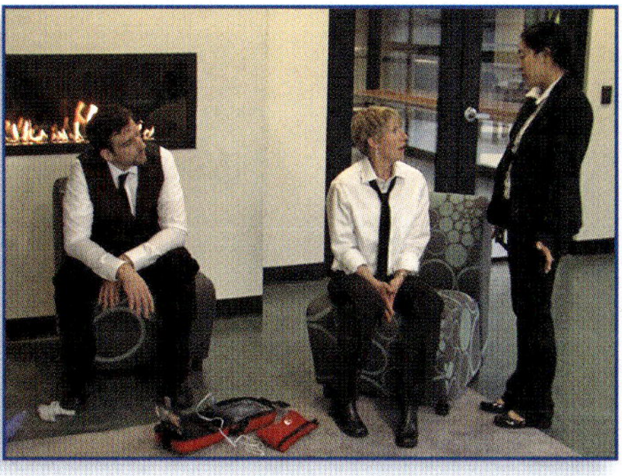

This is a normal human reaction to a traumatic event. Calm yourself as best you can and acknowledge your limitations as a provider.

When an emergency is over, a provider is often left alone while an ill or injured person is quickly transported away by EMS. With limited time for closure, you can begin to experience a variety of reactions. These may include the following:

- Feeling abandoned or helpless
- Recalling the event over and over
- Self-doubt about not doing enough

- Difficulty concentrating
- Heaviness in the chest
- Upset stomach or diarrhea
- Difficulty sleeping or nightmares

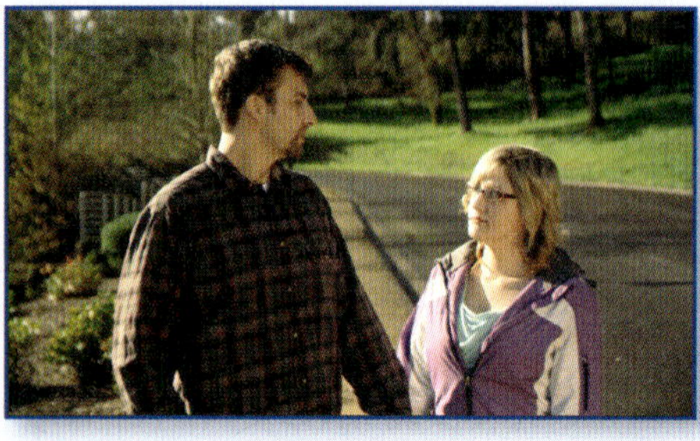

These feelings are normal and should pass with time. However, there are actions you can take to help work through the difficulty:

- Share your feelings.
- Talk with someone you trust to listen without judgment, such as a family member, friend, or coworker.
- Get back to a normal routine as soon as possible.
- Accept that it will take time to resolve these emotions.
- If unpleasant feelings persist, formal assistance from a professional counselor may be helpful as you deal with your emotions about the event.

Knowledge Check

You responded as a first aid provider to a coworker who experienced a life-threatening allergic reaction to a bee sting. She has been transported by EMS to a hospital for further care. The experience was overwhelming, and you still have not heard if her condition has improved. The experience has clearly left you shaken. You keep going over your actions in your head and wonder if you did enough. How can you help address the feelings you are having?

Glossary

abdominal thrust

Thrusts administered to the abdomen of a responsive, choking person to dislodge an object blocking a person's airway.

acute coronary syndrome (ACS)

Often described as a heart attack, ACS occurs when there is reduced blood flow to the tissues of the heart.

airway

The passageway between mouth and lungs that allows life-sustaining oxygen into the body.

altered mental status

A significant change in a person's personality, behavior, or consciousness, which may indicate a serious medical problem.

amputation

A complete loss of a body part.

anaphylaxis

A severe allergic reaction with an extreme response of the body's immune system to something it is very sensitive to.

arterial bleeding

A wound to an artery, which is characterized by bright red, oxygen-rich blood spurting from the wound.

asthma

Reactive airway disease, narrowing the small air passages in the lungs and causing difficulty in breathing.

automated external defibrillator (AED)

A small, portable, computerized device that allows a minimally trained bystander to provide defibrillation much faster than EMS.

bloodborne pathogens

Infectious microorganisms in human blood that can cause disease in humans. These pathogens include, hepatitis B (HBV), hepatitis C (HCV) and human immunodeficiency virus (HIV).

cardiopulmonary resuscitation (CPR)

A combination of rescue breaths and chest compressions performed on a person experiencing cardiac arrest, intended to restore some oxygen to the brain.

chain of survival

A concept of five interdependent links (early access to EMS, early CPR, rapid defibrillation, effective advanced care, and integrated post-cardiac care) that describe the most effective approach for treating sudden cardiac arrest.

chest compression

A basic CPR skill that creates increased pressure in the chest cavity and direct compression of the heart. This forces blood to move from the chest to the lungs, brain, and rest of the body.

chest thrust

Thrusts administered on the breastbone of a responsive, choking person to dislodge an object stuck in the person's airway.

compression-only CPR

A simple, but limited, approach to treating sudden cardiac arrest that is being widely promoted to people who are not formally trained in CPR.

CPR mask

A protective barrier device used to prevent exposure to potentially infectious body fluids while performing rescue breaths on a person. The mask fits over the mouth and nose of the person and includes a one-way valve to blow through.

defibrillation

The delivery of an electrical shock through the heart intended to end chaotic electrical activity in the heart and allow the heart's normal electrical activity to return.

diabetes

A disease in which the body cannot effectively use sugar for energy, which can lead to life-threatening problems if not managed properly. A diabetic emergency is often characterized by an altered mental status.

direct pressure

Pressure applied directly to a bleeding site until bleeding stops. It is the standard method for controlling external bleeding.

dislocation

The separation of bone ends at a joint.

DOTS

Mnemonic device used to help with physical assessment:

- Deformities
- Open injuries
- Tenderness
- Swelling

emergency action plan (EAP)

Used to help ensure safe and healthy conditions at work by provides step-by-step procedures on how to report and respond to emergencies.

emergency medical services (EMS)

An emergency medical response system developed within a community, consisting of a specialized communications network and trained professional responders, all accessible through an emergency phone number such as 911.

epinephrine auto-injector

A prescribed medication device with a spring-loaded needle, designed for easy use by a minimally trained person. Intended for use in treating a life-threatening allergic reaction, it delivers a measured single dose of epinephrine.

evisceration

The protrusion of abdominal organs through an open abdominal wound.

FAST

Mnemonic device used to help with stroke assessment:

- Face droop
- Arm drift
- Speech difficulty
- Time to activate EMS

fracture

A break in a bone.

frostbite

The freezing of skin and underlying body tissue in extremely cold conditions.

Good Samaritan law

A law enacted to legally protect trained providers who voluntarily stop to help, act prudently, do not provide care beyond training, and are not completely careless in delivering emergency care.

head tilt-chin lift

The recommended technique to open and maintain the airway of an unresponsive person. It pulls the jaw forward and lifts the tongue away from the back of the throat.

heart attack

See *acute coronary syndrome.*

hypoglycemia

Low blood sugar. A diabetic condition that can rapidly develop and become life threatening.

hypothermia

A generalized cooling of the body that is a life-threatening condition, occurring when the internal core body temperature has decreased to 95° F or less.

impaled object

An object that penetrates a body part and remains embedded.

implied consent

A legal concept referring to the assumption that an unresponsive person would give permission to be helped if responsive.

internal bleeding

A condition in which an injury causes bleeding inside the body, which can be difficult to detect. If it goes untreated, it can lead to shock and become a life-threatening problem.

mechanism of injury

A concept used by first aid providers to quickly suspect injury due to evidence that significant force has impacted a person's body.

naloxone

A medication that can temporarily reverse the life-threatening effects of opioids. It is administered either through an auto-injector device or through an aerosol that is sprayed into the nose. Naloxone is becoming more readily available to lay providers.

overlay shield

A protective barrier device used to prevent exposure to potentially infectious body fluids while performing rescue breaths on a person. The shield lays over the face and includes a one-way valve or filter to blow through.

primary assessment

An initial approach to quickly identify if a life-threatening condition is present.

protective barrier

An item that helps reduce the risk of exposure to blood and other potentially infectious body fluids. Examples include disposable gloves, CPR masks, and face shields.

recovery position

A side-lying position in which an unresponsive breathing person is placed to drain fluids from the mouth and keep the tongue from blocking the airway.

rescue breaths

Artificial breaths given to someone who is not breathing, administered by blowing air into the mouth to inflate the lungs.

SAMPLE

Mnemonic device used to help providers remember what to ask a person about:

- Symptoms
- Allergies
- Medications
- Past medical history
- Last oral intake
- Events leading to problem

secondary assessment

Used when there are no life-threatening conditions to gather additional information about the person's chief complaint, physical signs, and additional information related to what is going on.

seizure

Jerking or convulsive activity of the body triggered by excessive electrical activity within the brain.

shock

A life-threatening condition that develops when poor blood flow creates a shortage of oxygen to body tissues.

spinal motion restriction

The use of the hands to gently hold both sides of the head to restrict spinal. Done to prevent additional damage from a suspected spinal injury.

splint

A device used externally to immobilize a painful, swollen, or deformed limb in order to decrease pain and prevent further injury.

sprains

Tearing injuries to ligaments that hold joins together.

standard precautions

A consistent set of protective practices used whether or not an infection is suspected. The approach is the same for everyone, regardless of relationship or age.

strains

Stretching or tearing injuries to muscles or tendons.

stroke

Sudden brain cell death caused by the loss of oxygen to brain tissue either by a blockage in a blood vessel or bleeding into brain tissue when a weak blood vessel wall bursts open.

sudden cardiac arrest (SCA)

The abrupt loss of the heart's ability to contract and push blood forward through the circulatory system. Typically caused by a sudden disruption of the heart's electrical system.

tourniquet

A binding device used on a limb above a heavily bleeding wound to control bleeding.

unresponsive

A condition in which a person does not respond to physical or verbal attempts to get a response.

ventricular fibrillation

A chaotic, quivering heart rhythm that prevents the normal contraction of the heart and the ability to pump blood.

Sources

The MEDIC First Aid BasicPlus Student Book is based upon the following standards, guidelines, and recommendations:

2015 International Consensus on Cardiopulmonary Resuscitation and Emergency Cardiovascular Care Science With Treatment Recommendations. *Circulation* 132, suppl 1 (2015):S2–S268.

2015 International Consensus on First Aid Science With Treatment Recommendations. *Circulation* 132, suppl 1 (2015):S269–S311.

2015 American Heart Association Guidelines Update for Cardiopulmonary Resuscitation and Emergency Cardiovascular Care. *Circulation* 132, suppl 2 (2015):S315–S573.

2015 American Heart Association and American Red Cross Guidelines Update for First Aid. *Circulation* 132, suppl 2 (2015): S574–S589.

ANSI/ASSE. *Z490.1-2016: Criteria for Accepted Practices in Safety, Health, & Environmental Training Standard*. Park Ridge, IL: ASSE, 2016.

ASTM International. *F2171-02 Standard Guide for Defining the Performance of First Aid Providers in Occupational Settings*. West Conshohocken, PA: ASTM International, 2009.

U.S. Occupational Safety and Health Administration. *Best Practices Guide: Fundamentals of a Workplace First-Aid Program*. OSHA 3317-06N. Washington DC: Department of Labor, 2006.

ADDITIONAL INFORMATION

Endnotes

1. Centers for Disease Control and Prevention, National Hospital Ambulatory Medical Care Survey: 2011 Emergency Department Summary Tables, (2011), http://www.cdc.gov/nchs/data/ahcd/nhamcs_emergency/2011_ed_web_tables.pdf.

2. "Latex Allergy," *MedlinePlus Medical Encyclopedia*, U.S. National Library of Medicine, last updated March 9, 2016, https://www.nlm.nih.gov/medlineplus/latexallergy.html.

3. American Academy of Pediatrics, American Public Health Association, National Resource Center for Health and Safety in Child Care and Early Education. 2011. *Caring for our Children: National Health and Safety Performance Standards; Guidelines for Early Care and Education Programs. 3rd Edition.* Appendix J, P 441. Elk Grove Village, IL: American Academy of Pediatrics; Washington, DC: American Public Health Association.

4. "Anaphylaxis," *MedlinePlus Medical Encyclopedia*, U.S. National Library of Medicine, last updated May 11, 2014, https://www.nlm.nih.gov/medlineplus/ency/article/000844.htm.

5. James Mowry et al., "2014 Annual Report of the American Association of Poison Control Centers' National Poison Data System (NPDS): 32nd Annual Report." *Clinical Toxicology* 53, no. 10 (November 26, 2015): 962–1147. doi:10.3109/15563650.2015.1102927.

6. "Heat Emergencies," *MedlinePlus Medical Encyclopedia*, U.S. National Library of Medicine, last updated January 13, 2014, https://www.nlm.nih.gov/medlineplus/ency/article/000056.htm.

7. "Snake Bites," *MedlinePlus Medical Encyclopedia*, U.S. National Library of Medicine, last updated January 13, 2014, https://www.nlm.nih.gov/medlineplus/ency/article/000031.htm.

Knowledge Check Answers

Preparing to Help — *Page 3*

If the scene is safe, you should still approach and offer to help your coworker who was struck. You are only the first link in a progressive chain of emergency care. Your involvement lasts only until relieved by another first aid provider or responding EMS personnel — in most cases, a very short period of time. Your training provides you with sound knowledge and skills designed only to help — and not harm — those in need. Extensive medical knowledge is not necessary. First aid is simple and easy to provide.

Protecting Yourself — *Page 5*

False. Standard precautions is a set of protective practices used whether or not an infection is suspected. To be effective, your approach is the same for everyone, regardless of relationship or age.

Legal Considerations — *Page 8*

Implied consent, which assumes your coworker would agree to be helped given the circumstances, applies in this situation.

Calling for Help — *Page 11*

Yes. EMS activation is appropriate when there are immediate threats to life, a significant mechanism of injury has occurred, warning signs of serious illness exist, or if you are unsure about the severity of a person's condition.

Emergency Moves — *Page 12*

Using your legs, not your back, drag your coworker from the smoke-filled area to a safer location. It is best not to move an ill or injured person at all unless he or she is clearly endangered or requires life-supporting care, which is true in this case.

Cardiac Arrest — *Page 17*

1. Early recognition of cardiac arrest and activation of EMS
2. Immediate CPR with high-quality chest compressions
3. Rapid defibrillation, or electrical shock, to the heart with an AED

Chest Compressions — *Page 19*

1. Compress deeply, more than 2 inches
2. Compress fast, between 100 to 120 times per minute
3. Allow the chest wall to fully recoil, or rebound, between compressions. Avoid leaning on the chest at the top of each compression.

Rescue Breaths — *Page 23*

Each breath should be about 1 second in length, and only have enough air to create a visible rise of the chest, but no more. Additional air is unnecessary.

Automated External Defibrillation — *Page 29*

1. Turn on the AED.
2. Adhere defibrillation pads to bare chest.
3. Allow the AED to analyze the heart rhythm.
4. Deliver a shock if directed to by the AED.

Primary Assessment — Unresponsive Person — *Page 32*

Perform CPR immediately, starting with compressions. Irregular gasping, snorting, or gurgling sounds do not provide oxygen and do not indicate normal breathing.

Caring for Cardiac Arrest — *Page 37*

Begin CPR starting with compressions. Perform ongoing cycles of 30 chest compressions and 2 rescue breaths. Take no longer than 10 seconds to give the 2 rescue breaths. Stop CPR when the AED is attached and ready to analyze. Deliver a shock if advised by the AED. Immediately resume CPR.

Multiple Provider Approach to CPR — *Page 39*

Communicate about the switch ahead of time. Coordinate your actions to switch smoothly and minimize interruption time. Prior to the arrival of an AED, switch at the end of a CPR cycle, while the person who is going to move out is giving rescue breaths.

Choking — *Page 42*

Stand behind him. Reach around and locate his navel with your finger. Make a fist with your other hand and place the thumb side against the abdomen, just above your finger and below his ribs. Grasp your fist with the other hand and give a quick inward and upward thrust to expel the obstruction. Repeat thrusts until he can breathe normally.

Primary Assessment — Responsive Person — *Page 45*

If serious bleeding is found during a primary assessment, control it immediately. Do not continue the assessment.

Secondary Assessment — *Page 48*

A head to toe physical assessment using the DOTS mnemonic as a guide and questioning him using the SAMPLE mnemonic as a guide.

Control of Bleeding — *Page 51*

Pressure applied directly to a bleeding site until bleeding stops is the standard method for controlling external bleeding. If direct pressure is unable to control bleeding on a limb, use a tourniquet.

Shock — *Page 60*

Early signs of shock can be difficult to detect. A person may simply begin to appear uneasy, restless, or worried. Other, more serious signs can emerge gradually. The person may become confused. The skin may become pale, cool, and sweaty.

Amputation — *Page 61*

True. If an amputation has occurred, quickly assess for and control any severe bleeding. Once the person is stable, locate and manage the severed part.

Impaled Objects — *Page 63*

1. If it has damaged any large blood vessels, it can act like a plug, helping to prevent serious blood loss.
2. Movement of the object, or the body part it is in, could also create additional injury, especially if the object is embedded in muscle, bone, or organs below the skin.

Open Chest Injury — *Page 64*

False. Sealing an open chest wound with an airtight dressing could result in an increasing pressure within the chest which could quickly become life-threatening.

Open Abdominal Injury — *Page 65*

Cover any protruding organs with a thick, moist dressing. Do not push the organs back inside the body.

Head, Neck, and Back Injury — *Page 68*

The lack of symptoms or obvious injury does not mean that the spine is not injured. If a significant mechanism of injury occurred, it is best to assume a spinal injury exists.

Swollen, Painful, Deformed Limb — *Page 71*

It is best to not straighten an injured limb that is unnaturally angled. Leave the limb in the position found. If a limb becomes blue or extremely pale, circulation may be compromised by the injury. Activate EMS if this occurs.

Burns — *Page 76*

Cool a burn with cool or cold water as quickly as possible and for at least 10 minutes.

Minor Injuries — *Page 78*

When a tooth has been knocked out, treat it without delay. Immediate reimplantation is believed by the dental community to result in the greatest chance of tooth survival.

Altered Mental Status — *Page 84*

If uninjured, place the person in a recovery position.

Breathing Difficulty or Shortness of Breath — *Page 86*

Breathing difficulty can quickly become life-threatening as a person becomes exhausted from the breathing effort. Be prepared to provide CPR and attach an AED if breathing stops.

Pain, Pressure, or Discomfort in the Chest — *Page 88*

True. This is a common occurrence in this situation. Accept it, but never let this alter your approach to care.

Poisoning — *Page 91*

1-800-222-1222

Severe Abdominal Pain — *Page 93*

A person complaining of severe abdominal pain will typically try to find a position of comfort, often with the knees raised, to relieve the pain. Help the person to maintain this position.

Heat Emergencies — *Page 96*

Activate EMS immediately. The most important action a first aid provider can take is to begin immediate cooling with the resources available. When possible, the best method for cooling is to immerse the person up to the chin in cold water.

Cold Emergencies — *Page 99*

Hypothermia, a generalized cooling of the body.

Stinging Insects — *Page 101*

Remove the stinger quickly as possible. It may still be injecting venom into her body.

Snakebites — *Page 103*

Venomous cottonmouths, copperheads, and rattlesnakes are known as pit vipers. Pit vipers strike once and leave a characteristic bite with single or double fang mark.

Spider Bites — *Page 104*

Over time, cramping pain and muscular rigidity in the body may occur. A person may experience fever, weakness, nausea and vomiting, or difficulty breathing.

Tick Bites — *Page 105*

The exposure and transmission of infectious disease, most notably Lyme disease.

Marine Animal Stings — *Page 107*

1. Wash the sting site liberally with household vinegar as soon as possible for at least 30 seconds to deactivate the venom and prevent further stinging.
2. To help reduce pain, shower or immerse the sting site with hot water for at least 20 minutes or until the pain subsides.

Animal and Human Bites — *Page 108*

There is concern for rabies, which is fatal if left untreated.

Emotional Considerations — *Page 110*

It is normal to feel anxious and emotional following an emergency. Try to share your feelings with someone you trust. If possible, return to your normal routine, and give yourself time to resolve your emotions about the experience. If your unpleasant feelings persist, consider seeing a professional counselor.

Rate Your Program

This course evaluation allows you to rate the training course you have just completed. This evaluation will provide your training provider with feedback on the quality of the instruction you received.

Program Name________________________ ☐ ASHI ☐ MEDIC First Aid

Instructor ________________________ Date of Course__________

Please rate the following course elements as indicated below. Place a check in the box that best represents your opinion of the quality of each element. *Thank you for your help.*	4–Excellent	3–Good	2–Average	1–Poor
Course Presentation				
Organization, pace, and flow	☐	☐	☐	☐
Not too basic, not too complex	☐	☐	☐	☐
Time allowed for skill practice	☐	☐	☐	☐
Increased your confidence and ability to take action	☐	☐	☐	☐
Instructor(s)				
Subject knowledge	☐	☐	☐	☐
Teaching ability (clear, concise, organized)	☐	☐	☐	☐
Demeanor (friendly, helpful, engaging)	☐	☐	☐	☐
Program Materials				
Video	☐	☐	☐	☐
PowerPoint®	☐	☐	☐	☐
Student Book	☐	☐	☐	☐
Online Training Component (if taken)	☐	☐	☐	☐
Location and Equipment				
Space	☐	☐	☐	☐
Training equipment	☐	☐	☐	☐
Self Assessment				
How would you rate your emergency care skills BEFORE taking this class?	☐	☐	☐	☐
How would you rate your emergency care skills AFTER taking this class?	☐	☐	☐	☐
How willing would you be to respond in an emergency BEFORE taking this class?	☐	☐	☐	☐
How willing would you be to respond in an emergency AFTER taking this class?	☐	☐	☐	☐
Your overall score for the course	☐	☐	☐	☐

What did you like most about this course? ________________________

____

What did you like least about this course? ________________________

____

Would you recommend this course to others? ☐ Yes ☐ No

Student input is an essential aspect of our ongoing quality assurance efforts. HSI requires that students be given the opportunity to evaluate their ASHI or MEDIC First Aid course using this "Rate Your Program" course evaluation form. You also may provide feedback directly to HSI at www.hsi.com/rateyourprogram.